T0292701

CAMBRIDGE LIBRARY COLLECTION

Books of enduring scholarly value

History of Medicine

It is sobering to realise that as recently as the year in which On the Origin of Species was published, learned opinion was that diseases such as typhus and cholera were spread by a 'miasma', and suggestions that doctors should wash their hands before examining patients were greeted with mockery by the profession. The Cambridge Library Collection reissues milestone publications in the history of Western medicine as well as studies of other medical traditions. Its coverage ranges from Galen on anatomical procedures to Florence Nightingale's common-sense advice to nurses, and includes early research into genetics and mental health, colonial reports on tropical diseases, documents on public health and military medicine, and publications on spa culture and medicinal plants.

Essays Medical and Experimental

A physician and medical reformer enthused by the scientific and cultural progress of the Enlightenment as it took hold in Britain, Thomas Percival (1740–1804) wrote on many topics, including public health and demography. His influential *Medical Ethics* (also reissued in this series) is considered the first modern formulation. This one-volume reissue brings together two volumes of his essays on a variety of medical subjects, published in a revised second edition of 1772 and a follow-up collection of 1773. Many of the essays reflect his concern for public health, particularly for the citizens of Manchester. The appendix to the first volume includes two essays that were previously unpublished. Several of the pieces record medical oddities encountered by Percival, and others document his observations on the possible medicinal applications of certain plants, including coffee. His four-volume *Works* (1807), containing additional essays that appeared after 1773, is also reissued in this series.

Cambridge University Press has long been a pioneer in the reissuing of out-of-print titles from its own backlist, producing digital reprints of books that are still sought after by scholars and students but could not be reprinted economically using traditional technology. The Cambridge Library Collection extends this activity to a wider range of books which are still of importance to researchers and professionals, either for the source material they contain, or as landmarks in the history of their academic discipline.

Drawing from the world-renowned collections in the Cambridge University Library and other partner libraries, and guided by the advice of experts in each subject area, Cambridge University Press is using state-of-the-art scanning machines in its own Printing House to capture the content of each book selected for inclusion. The files are processed to give a consistently clear, crisp image, and the books finished to the high quality standard for which the Press is recognised around the world. The latest print-on-demand technology ensures that the books will remain available indefinitely, and that orders for single or multiple copies can quickly be supplied.

The Cambridge Library Collection brings back to life books of enduring scholarly value (including out-of-copyright works originally issued by other publishers) across a wide range of disciplines in the humanities and social sciences and in science and technology.

Essays Medical and Experimental

The Second Edition, Revised, and Considerably Enlarged. To Which is Added an Appendix

Thomas Percival

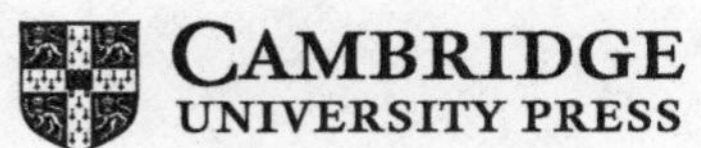

CAMBRIDGE
UNIVERSITY PRESS

University Printing House, Cambridge, CB2 8BS, United Kingdom

Published in the United States of America by Cambridge University Press, New York

Cambridge University Press is part of the University of Cambridge.
It furthers the University's mission by disseminating knowledge in the pursuit of education, learning and research at the highest international levels of excellence.

www.cambridge.org
Information on this title: www.cambridge.org/9781108067935

This edition first published 1772–3
This digitally printed version 2014

ISBN 978-1-108-06793-5 Paperback

ESSAYS

MEDICAL

AND

EXPERIMENTAL.

ESSAYS

MEDICAL

AND

EXPERIMENTAL.

THE SECOND EDITION,

REVISED, AND CONSIDERABLY ENLARGED.

TO WHICH IS ADDED AN

APPENDIX.

BY

THOMAS PERCIVAL, M.D. F.R.S.

——— *Relinquamus aliquid quo nos vixisse testemur.*

Plin. Epist. Lib. 3. Ep. 7.

LONDON:

Printed for J. JOHNSON, No. 72, St. Paul's Church-Yard.

MDCCLXXII.

Quantacunque fuerint aliorum conamina, ſemper exiſtimavi mihi vitalis auræ uſum fruſtra datum fore, niſi et ipſe, in hoc ſtudio verſatus, ſymbolum aliquod, utcunque exiguum, in commune medicinæ ærarium contribuerem.

SYDENHAM.

TO

Thomas Butterworth Bayley, Efq;

Of HOPE,

Near MANCHESTER.

ACCEPT, dear Sir, this tribute of efteem, refpect, and affection; and whilft I am difcharging the debt of juftice to fuperiour abilities, active virtue, and the moft amiable manners, allow me the honour of being known

known to the world as the friend of Mr. BAYLEY, and of ſubſcribing myſelf,

DEAR SIR,

Your faithful, affectionate,

and moſt obedient Servant,

MANCHESTER,
1ſt *Decem.* 1771.

THOMAS PERCIVAL.

THE

PREFACE.

THE Author of the following Eſſays, preſuming on the candid reception which they met with from the public, commits to the ſame indulgence, the preſent enlarged and improved edition of them. The firſt and ſecond Diſſertations, which are the productions of his youth, illuſtrate both the inſufficiency of theory, and the danger of truſt-

ing

ing to experience alone in the practice of physic. The annals of medicine abound with instances of the fatal effects of Empiricism, and Hypothetical reasoning, founded on fictitious principles. But these examples, painful as they are to a feeling mind, impeach not the honour or usefulness of the healing art; and are chargeable only on the ignorance of a few of its professors, and on the credulity of mankind. The History of the Christian Church presents us with a picture still more shocking to humanity: But who disputes the influence of religion, to promote the peace, order, and happiness of society, because superstition hath occasioned so much confusion, misery,

misery, and devastation? It is seriously to be lamented that juster ideas are not formed of the nature, extent, and objects of medicine in general; and of the several branches, into which as a practical science, too comprehensive for any individual to exercise, it is now divided. This would prevent the encouragement of illiterate pretenders; would conciliate harmony, and excite a generous emulation amongst the different orders of the faculty; and by confining the exertions of each, within the sphere adapted to their genius and education, would powerfully promote the improvement of Physic, Surgery, and Pharmacy. No profession requires a more enlarged and cultivated

cultivated underſtanding, or comprehends a wider circle of knowledge than that of phyſic. And to the honour of the Phyſicians of this age and country it may with truth be aſſerted, that they are peculiarly diſtinguiſhed as men of liberal education, and extenſive learning. *(a)*

THE third Eſſay conſiſts of experiments and obſervations on Bitters and Aſtringents in general, and on the Peruvian Bark in particular. The utility of this method of

(a) MR. JUSTICE BLACKSTONE recommends the ſtudy of the law, to gentlemen of the faculty of phyſic, with this honourable diſtinction, "to compleat the character of general and extenſive knowledge; a character which their profeſſion, beyond others, has remarkably deſerved." Blackſtone's Comment. Vol. 1. p. 14.

of inquiry is univerſally acknowledged; and nothing can tend more to the advancement of real ſcience, than the ſteady purſuit of it. The improvements which have been made in the art of medicine for this century paſt, are more than equal to thoſe of a thouſand preceding years. And theſe improvements may be juſtly aſcribed to that taſte for experiment which hath of late ſo generally prevailed. But though much hath been done in this way of inveſtigation, there are ſtill numberleſs untrodden paths in Phyſic which remain to be explored. And every perſon of tolerable abilities, who hath patience, aſſiduity, and a ſufficient minuteneſs of attention, may almoſt aſſure himſelf

himſelf that his labours will be rewarded with ſucceſs, and that he can hardly fail of adding ſome new and uſeful diſcoveries to the common ſtock of medical knowledge. *Multum egerunt qui ante nos fuerunt, ſed non peregerunt ; multum adhuc reſtat operæ, multumq; reſtabit, neque ulli nato poſt mille ſecula præcidetur occaſio aliquid adhuc adjiciendi. (a)* The Author might have confirmed many of the obſervations contained in this Eſſay by a variety of experiments, which he has lately made on the Columbo Root ; a medicine, which from its efficacy, deſerves to be more generally known in practice. But his papers on that ſubject are laid before

(a) Seneca.

fore the Royal Society, and will probably be publiſhed in the next Volume of Philoſophical Tranſactions. *(a)*

THE title of the fourth Eſſay fully explains the purport of it. An attempt to aſcertain the uſe and operation of a remedy ſo well known as Bliſters, may at firſt view appear to be unneceſſary. But a more attentive examination will convince us of our miſtake. The

(a) THE Columbo Root is cordial, corroborant, antiſeptic, and powerfully antiemetic. It is a uſeful remedy in the cholera morbus; in diarrhœas; in the dyſentery; in bilious fevers; in a languid ſtate of the ſtomach, attended with want of appetite, nauſea, and indigeſtion; and in habitual vomitings, when they proceed from a weakneſs or irritability of the ſtomach, from an irregular gout, from acidities, or from acrimonious bile. Experience confirms the truth of theſe obſervations, and the following facts ſerve in ſome meaſure to explain them. An

The triteneſs of the ſubject is the reaſon that it has been ſo much overlooked and neglected; and though veſicatories are employed and recommended by almoſt every medical practitioner, yet few have attended to their real action, or to the general principles which ought to direct their application.

THE ſubject of the fifth Eſſay, the author confeſſes, is rather curious than uſeful, of more importance to the inquiſitive phyſiologiſt,

An infuſion of the Columbo Root mixes uniformly with putrid bile, and inſtantly corrects the fœtor of it; preſerves freſh bile from putrefaction conſiderably longer than moſt other antiſeptics; moderates without ſuſpending the fermentation of alimentary mixtures; prevents them from growing ſour; and neutraliſes acidities when formed, much more compleatly than Peruvian bark or chamomile flowers.—The virtues of this Root are extracted both by water and rectified ſpirit of wine, and by cold maceration, as well as by decoction, or infuſion with heat.

logiſt, than to the practical phyſician. But as all reſearches into the operations of nature merit our notice and regard, an inquiry into the reſemblance between the Chyle and Milk hath certainly ſome claim to our attention. And if it appear probable, as he preſumes it will, that Milk is the Chyle unaſſimilated, or at leaſt very little changed, it may lead to ſome uſeful inferences concerning the proper diet for nurſes.

THE two firſt tracts contained in the Appendix were publiſhed ſeparately a few years ago; and as no copies of the former impreſſion now remain, they are reprinted and annexed, not improperly it is hoped, to this Volume of Eſſays.

THE

THE Obſervations on the efficacy of external applications in the Ulcerous Sore Throat were written in the ſummer of 1770, a period when that diſeaſe was epidemical in the town and neighbourhood of Mancheſter. The meaſles alſo prevailed very generally at the ſame time; but though theſe diſorders have been often obſerved to aſſociate themſelves together, and may ſeem to bear ſome analogy to each other, from the efflo-reſcence on the ſkin, and inflammation of the eyes, with which they are both accompanied, no inſtance then occurred to the Author of their union.

ESSAY I.

THE

EMPIRIC;

OR,

ARGUMENTS AGAINST THE USE

OF

THEORY AND REASONING

IN PHYSIC.

Sufficit ſi quid fiat intelligamus, etiamſi quomodo quidque fiat ignoremus.

CICERO.

Non fingendum ant excogitandum, ſed inveniendum quid natura faciat aut ferat.

BACON.

ESSAY I.

THE EMPIRIC; OR, MAN OF EXPERIENCE. (a)

IN this polished age, when every art is advancing towards perfection, and every science enlarging its boundaries, it is a melancholy consideration that MEDICINE should alone be left behind in

(a) THIS and the following dissertation contain a discussion of the arguments for and against the use of theory and reasoning in medicine. They are not intended as an explanation of the tenets of those two ancient and celebrated sects of physicians, the Empirics and Rationalists, of which Celsus hath given us so elegant an

in the general career of improvement. The miſts of ignorance and error are now vaniſhing before the lights of genuine philoſophy; and knowledge, practical and ſpeculative, extends its influence even to the meaneſt mechanic. But the Hippocratic art, amidſt this rapid and almoſt univerſal revolution, is at leaſt ſtationary, if it move not in a retrograde courſe. And what is ſingular in its fate, the ſame cauſes which have promoted the advancement of the ſiſter ſciences, have by a wrong direction checked the growth, and

an account; but to point out opinions which now prevail in the world, and which naturally ariſe from the different lights, in which the ſame ſubject is viewed by different minds. The author hath endeavoured to ſuppoſe himſelf firſt of the one party, and then of the other; in order more fully to enter into the ſentiments of each, and by that means do juſtice to both ſides of the queſtion. In this kind of writing it is not eaſy to avoid declamation; and he hopes to be excuſed, if he has indulged ſome degree of that enthuſiaſm, with which two antagoniſts may be ſuppoſed to be actuated, when pleading againſt each other, in ſupport of a favourite cauſe.

and retarded the progreſs of one which is

—— fairly worth the ſeven.

POPE.

THE induſtry of its profeſſors, by an injudicious application, hath ſerved only to darken and perplex it. Inſtead of patiently treading in the ſure ſteps of EXPERIENCE, they have followed the falſe clue of THEORY; and whilſt with infinite pains and labour they endeavour to penetrate into the receſſes of phyſic, they have loſt themſelves in the labyrinths of error. Unhappily for the healing art, their miſtakes have coincided with the common propenſities of mankind, who are more inclined to ſearch after hidden and undiſcoverable cauſes, than to attend to the obvious phœnomena of nature. Blinded with their own fictions, theſe wanton theoriſts conceal their ignorance from themſelves and the world, by unmeaning terms and pompous phraſes.

"*Omnia enim ſtolidi magis admirantur amantque*
"*Inverſis quæ ſub verbis latitantia cernunt.*"
LUCRETIUS.

BUT deſcending from the flights of declamation, let us point out the folly, detect the fallacy, and trace the dangerous conſequences of theory and reaſoning in medicine.

WHOEVER ſearches into the annals of phyſic cannot fail of being aſtoniſhed at the almoſt infinite variety of ſyſtems and hypotheſes, which at different times have been obtruded on the world. The amazing fertility of the imagination is there diſplayed in its full extent; and perhaps ſo ample an exhibition of the powers of human invention might gratify the vanity of man, if the agreeable effect were

were not more than counter-balanced by the humbling view of ſo much abſurdity, contradiction, and falſhood. The idleſt opinions have had their abettors; the moſt groundleſs fictions have been ſwallowed with credulity. A liſt of all the follies which at different periods have been eſtabliſhed as articles of faith in medicine, would form the ſevereſt ſatyr on the healing art. Who can withold his laughter when he reads of expelling, attracting, and concocting faculties; of energies, ſympathies, antipathies, idioſyncraſies, and occult cauſes; of the body being nothing but ſalt, ſulphur, and mercury; of man being a microcoſm, and uniting in his frame the motion of the ſtars, the nature of the earth, of water, air, all vegetables and minerals, the conſtellations, and the four winds. Yet ridiculous as theſe ſeveral tenets may appear, they have given riſe to ſects, have been eſpouſed with warmth, and defended with acrimony. But the excentric genius of the theorifts hath not been confined within the limits of phyfiology, and the laws of the animal œconomy: the hidden caufes of difeafes, the elements or firft principles of medicines, and their fecret mode of action on the body, have afforded another no lefs extenfive field for the exercife of their creative imaginations. The bare recital of their fictions, would fufficiently demonftrate their abfurdity. But to enumerate them would be an almoft endlefs tafk. Erafiftratus defines difeafe to be a tranflation of blood from the veins to the arteries; whereas Galen afferts that as health confifts in the equilibrium between drynefs and moifture, heat and cold; ficknefs muft depend upon the fubverfion of that equilibrium. One fect adopts *plethora* as the caufe of all difeafes; another denies the poffibility of its exiftence in the body. Sylvius exults in the difcovery that an acid is the fole morbid principle; his antagonifts afcribe that honour

honour to their alkali. Salt, ſulphur, acrimonies, cauſtics, volatiles, ferments, &c. &c. have each at different times and by different ſyſtematics been received as the undoubted *principia morborum*. No leſs abſurd are the fictions of the theoriſts concerning the elements and qualities of medicines, and their operation on the body. The ſame drug is repreſented as hot in one degree and cold in another, or as dry in one proportion and moiſt in another. Certain remedies are whimſically aſſigned to particular parts of the body, on which they are ſuppoſed to exert their effects by a peculiar predilection. Hence the claſſes of pectorals, ſtomachics, hepatics, cephalics, cordials, &c. One medicine attracts and eliminates the bile, another the *pituita*, and a third the *atra bilis* or melancholy. Some preparations *irradiate* the animal ſpirits, others *darken* and *obſcure* them. But enough of theſe idle conceits, the offſpring

ſpring of theory, and the diſgrace of phyſic.

PERHAPS it may be objected, that though many vain and groundleſs hypotheſes have been advanced, there are two which will bear the teſt of ridicule, and which have had the ſuffrages of the wiſeſt and moſt learned men in their favour. Let us briefly examine their pretenſions to credibility.

1. GEORGE ERNEST STAHL, a German phyſician, of a ſubtil and metaphyſical genius, ſuppoſes two oppoſite principles or propenſities in the human frame; one conſtantly and uniformly tending to corruption and decay, the other to life and health. The former is founded on the elementary compoſition of the body, the latter depends on the power and energy of the mind. By means of the nerves, the influence of the mind is extended to every part of the ſyſtem, and if

if their action be impeded, disease is the unavoidable consequence. A superabundance and spissitude of the blood is therefore the proximate cause of sickness, as the energy of the mind is thereby diminished, and its action on the body obstructed. Hence to lessen the quantity, and break down the lentor of the blood, the soul exerts all its powers and excites hemorrhages, sweats, diarrhæas, fevers, and the like. Dr. Potterfield and Dr. Nichols have carried this theory still further. The latter in his prælection *de anima medica*, affirms without reserve, that the soul at first forms the body and afterwards governs it, that she regulates and conducts all its vital and natural motions, circulates the fluids and distributes them to the different parts of the system, with such velocity and in such proportion as she judges right, and that whenever the body is disordered, she excites those conflicts and commotions which are best adapted

adapted to reſtore it to health and ſoundneſs.

SUCH are the principles of the Stahlians. —Let the unprejudiced judge whether they need a ſerious refutation. Could a mariner plan and conſtruct a ſhip, launch it into the wide ocean, govern it in ſtorms, direct it from ſhoals and rocks, and ſteer it ſafe into the deſtined harbour, without being conſcious of the ſkill he exerts, and the labour he employs? The analogy is obvious; and it would be equally abſurd to ſuppoſe that the mind could form the body, regulate all its motions, ſuperintend its health, reſcue it from diſeaſe, and be perpetually occupied in planning and executing the wiſeſt deſigns, without the leaſt knowledge or conſciouſneſs of the power and energy ſhe every moment exerts.

BUT the firſt propoſition of the Stahlians confutes itſelf. For if the body and mind with equal force be conſtantly and uniformly tending different ways, no change can poſſibly enſue; agreeable to the well known axiom in phyſics, that action and reaction are equal, and deſtroy each other's effect. Not to inſiſt however on this error in philoſophy, the doctrine of the Stahlians in confining all diſeaſes to *lentor* and *plethora* is falſe and abſurd. The dropſy, ſcurvy, *cacochymia*, *pthiſis pulmonalis*, putrid fevers, and many of the nervous claſs of ailments, are accompanied for the moſt part with a thin and colliquated ſtate of the fluids. Nor is there more truth in the aſſertion, that every diſtemper is an effort of the mind to relieve the body. The ſlighteſt laceration of a tendon has been ſucceeded by the locked jaw, convulſions, and death. An indolent glandular tumour terminates not unfrequently in a cancer. A neglect to evacuate the bladder in due time hath occaſioned a ſuppreſſion of urine; and the palſy has been

been the conſequence of a profuſe hemorrhage. Are theſe then the wiſe conflicts of the ſoul to reſcue her ſuffering partner from impending evil! and muſt we view in the ſame light the *angina maligna*, the *tuſſis convulſiva*, the ſpaſmodic cholic, the *tetanus*, *catalepſis*, worms, rickets, &c. &c. No one but a theoriſt, blinded with the miſts of his own brain, would anſwer in the affirmative.

2. THE important diſcovery of the circulation of the blood in the beginning of the laſt century by the ever memorable Dr. Harvey, gave riſe to the introduction of MECHANICS into medicine. And as that ſyſtem of philoſophy was founded on the general laws of nature, it was obvious to infer its application to the human body; which was ſuppoſed to differ only from the univerſe of things, in the wonderful variety and complication of its machinery. Bellini, Borelli, Pitcairn, Keil

Keil and Boerhaave are the great ſupporters of this theory. According to the deſcription of the latter, the body is chiefly compoſed of a conic, elaſtic, inflected canal, divided into ſimilar leſſer ones proceeding from the ſame trunk, which being at laſt collected into a retiform contexture, mutually open into each other, and ſend off two orders of veſſels, lymphatics and veins, the one terminating in different cavities of the body, the other in the heart. Theſe tubes are deſtined for the conveyance of the animal fluids; in the circulation of which life conſiſts, and on whoſe free and undiſturbed motion health depends. *Obſtruction* therefore is the proximate cauſe of moſt diſeaſes. And as it is produced either by a conſtriction of the veſſels, or by a *lentor* in the blood, theſe are conſidered as the remote cauſes.

HOWEVER plauſible this theory may appear to be at firſt ſight, it will be found on on a ſtricter examination to be fallacious and defective. The mathematician who calculates the projectile force of the heart, the velocity of the blood in the arteries and the various ſecretions of the glands, from the known laws of fluids in motion, and the nature of tubes of different ſhapes and ſizes, muſt unavoidably be expoſed to a thouſand miſtakes. The veſſels of the body are too numerous and minute to admit of an accurate menſuration; and they are perhaps every moment undergoing changes from the diverſified action of that vital power which animates our wonderful ſyſtem. Hence ariſes the contrariety in the computations of philoſophers on this ſubject. Borelli reckons the reſiſtance which the heart overcomes in propelling the blood through the arteries and veins to be equal to 180000 pounds weight: Dr. Hales makes it amount to no more than 51 pounds; and Keil, though he computes the fluids of the human body to be five times more in quantity

quantity than Borelli ſuppoſes, hath reduced the ſum to a ſingle pound. One aſſerts that the preſſure of air, overcome in ordinary reſpiration, is equivalent to the weight of 14000 pounds; a ſecond proves it to be equal only to a 100 pounds; and a third makes it ſo inconſiderable, as to be almoſt below compariſon; whilſt all the three appeal to mathematical demonſtration. A ſimilar diverſity appears in the concluſions of the mathematicians, concerning the quantity of bile ſeparated by the liver. To determine this point, Borelli firſt meaſures the diameter of the *ductus communis choledochus*, which he finds to be the 225th part of the diameter of the *vena cava*, juſt before it enters the right auricle of the heart. Hence he infers that if 7680 pounds of blood (ſuppoſing the whole maſs to be twenty pounds, and to circulate ſixteen times every hour) paſſes through the *vena cava* in twenty four hours, the 225th part of this quantity, i. e.

thirty four pounds of bile muſt in the ſame ſpace of time be tranſmitted through the hepatic ducts: a concluſion altogether repugnant to fact and experience. And it will appear to be much more ſo, if we admit, with the later mathematicians, that the veſſels of the human body contain at a medium thirty pounds of blood; for then the quantity of bile, according to Borelli's method of reaſoning, muſt amount to eighty five pounds in one day. But in this, as in the former inſtance, Keil widely differs from Borelli, and with greater probability concludes that two drachms of bile and no more, are hourly ſeparated from the liver. In theſe calculations no attention is paid to the peculiar nature of the animal fluids. Water and wine, a poiſonous and wholeſome liquid, are governed by the ſame hydraulic laws, but their effects when circulating in the body would certainly be very different. We know from experience that the velocity of the pulſe is influenced

by

by the ſtate of the blood. Even the acceſſion of new chyle after each meal, quickens the action of the heart and arteries. The human body therefore is not to be conſidered as a mere machine; and that theory which is built on this foundation is evidently fallacious. (a)

BUT the mechanic hypotheſis is alſo inadequate and defective; for the animal frame is incident to numberleſs diſeaſes which have no dependence on obſtruction. The *morbi fibræ debilis et laxæ* are not even by Boerhaave himſelf aſcribed to this cauſe. The dropſy, ſcurvy, putrid fevers, ſmall-pox, meaſles, and *lues venerea,* are inexplicable on mechanical principles. The

(a) In the Philoſophical Tranſactions there is a table in which the ſeveral purgatives and emetics commonly in uſe are enumerated and adjuſted by mathematical rules to all ages, ſexes, and conſtitutions. The doſes of the medicines are as the ſquares of the conſtitutions. And in the Edinburgh Medical Eſſays there is a formal attempt to correct the errors of this table.

The *hydrophobia* ſeems to be entirely a nervous affection, and cannot with the leaſt propriety be ſuppoſed to ariſe from obſtruction. No inflammation is obſervable on diſſection in the fauces or gullet; nor is there any palſy in the muſcles ſubſervient to deglutition. A numerous claſs of diſeaſes depend upon that ſympathetic connexion which ſubſiſts between different parts of the body. When the ſtomach is out of order, languor, debility, watchfulneſs, the night mare, and ſometimes a *cephalæa, vertigo*, or *hemicrania* are the conſequences. A rough bone ſtimulating the nerves of the great toe, hath produced epileptic fits. And it is well known that children from the irritation of the gums in dentition are liable to vomiting, purging, fever, and convulſions. Theſe few inſtances are ſufficient to ſhew that the body is unhappily ſubject to many diſorders, beſides thoſe which proceed from obſtruction. And perhaps the concluſion may be carried

ſtill

ſtill further, when we conſider that in the operation for the aneuriſm a large artery is tied up, and the circulation of the blood for ſome time almoſt totally ſuppreſſed in the part, without any material injury to health. Morgagni relates that Valſalva affixed two ligatures to the carotids of a dog, who lived above twenty days after the operation, and might have continued longer if he had not been killed for the purpoſe of diſſection. Is it then to be ſuppoſed that the obſtruction of a few capillaries, which are united together by an infinite number of anaſtomoſing branches, can be productive of ſuch fatal conſequences, whilſt the courſe of the blood is ſtopped in large veſſels with impunity? Equally falſe and abſurd is the mechanical hypotheſis concerning the operation of medicines, which is ſuppoſed to depend upon the ſize, figure, and gravity of their conſtituent particles. Thus chalybeates, for example, are recommended in obſtructions of the *catamenia*, on account of the *momentum* which they communicate to the blood. And on the ſame principles, mercury is ſaid to break down the texture, and produce a colliquation of the animal fluids. But both theſe explanations however elegant in theory, are falſe in fact. From the experiments of the late Dr. Wright *(a)* it is evident that ſteel never enters the lacteals, and that it exerts its effects ſolely on the ſtomach and bowels. And it is ſurely beyond the bounds of credibility to ſuppoſe, that a grain or two of corroſive ſublimate, which is light enough to be ſuſpended and diſſolved in brandy, is capable, by its extraordinary weight, of diſſolving the *craſſamentum* of the blood. But it is the genius of theory to dignify trifles, and to aſcribe the moſt wonderful effects to the moſt inſignificant cauſes.

HAPPY however had it been for the world,

(a) Phil. Tranſ. Vol. 50. pt. 2. p. 595.

world, if the medical ſyſtems which have been obtruded on it were only chargeable with inutility, abſurdity, or falſehood. But alas! they have miſled the underſtanding, perverted the judgment, and given riſe to the moſt dangerous and fatal errors in practice. A ſhort view of the hiſtory of phyſick will convince us of this melancholy truth. The divine Hippocrates knew how to diſtinguiſh between theory and experience; and he ſuffered not his doctrines of fire and water, his elements with their powers, nature with its inclinations, averſions, attractions, repulſions, and ratiocinations, to influence his treatment of diſeaſes. But the conduct of his ſucceſſors was widely different.

ERASISTRATUS reaſoning on falſe and precarious principles, and neglecting experience, the ſole teſt of utility, proſcribes the uſe of venæſection and purging, and condemns them as remedies equally infamous and dangerous.

ASCLEPIADES, from whom the modern ſect of mechanics have borrowed many of their doctrines, ſuppoſing that health depends on the juſt proportion between the pores of the body and certain corpuſcles they are deſtined to receive and tranſmit, and that it is impaired whenever theſe corpuſcles are obſtructed in their paſſage, orders exerciſe on horſeback in the moſt ardent fevers. He advances it as a maxim, that one fever is to be cured by raiſing another; and that the ſtrength of the patient is to be exhauſted by watching and the endurance of thirſt. And his practice was ſtrictly and ſeverely conformable to his principles; for he would not allow the ſick to cool their mouths with a drop of water during the two firſt days of the diſorder. But he indulged his phrenitic patients in the uſe of wine, even to intoxication.

THEMISON, the diſciple of Aſclepiades, rejected

rejected some of the opinions of his master, and founded a new sect called the Methodics. But his practice did not materially differ from that of Asclepiades, and his success is recorded by Juvenal in the following line.

" *Quot Themison ægros autumno occiderit uno.*

GALEN for the most part followed the plan of Hippocrates in the treatment of diseases. But as the *materia medica* in the course of five hundred years had been much augmented, the prescriptions of Galen were devoid of the Hippocratic simplicity. And it is more than probable that his false and ridiculous theory concerning the primary qualities of hot and cold, dry and moist, led him into dangerous errors in the composition of medicines.

ORIBASIUS, Ætius, Alexander Trallianus, Paulus Ægineta, and their successors the

the Arabian physicians, attempted no material innovations, but humbly trod in the footsteps of Galen. The Arabians indeed introduced several new and valuable medicines into practice, such as manna, senna, tamarinds, cassia, and rhubarb. And by the cultivation of chemistry, they laid a foundation for the greatest and most important revolutions in the art of medicine. I omit the mention of Albertus Magnus, Arnoldus de Villa Nova, Raymund Lully, Johannes de Rupescissa, Isaac and John Hollandus, and Basil Valentine, who were all chemists, many of them inventors of *panaceas*, and probably the authors of much mischief. In the beginning of the sixteenth century, Paracelsus a native of Switzerland stood forth, and with matchless arrogance, and the most supercilious contempt of others, proclaimed his opinions to the world. Seated in his Professorial chair at Basil, he solemnly burnt the writings of Galen and Avicenna, intending to become himself, the sole oracle

oracle in phyſick. But his theory is wild, romantic, abſurd, and dangerous; a ridiculous mixture of magic, aſtrology, and chemiſtry. The body he ſays, is compoſed of ſalt, ſulphur, and mercury; and in theſe three firſt ſubſtances, as he terms them, health and diſeaſes conſiſt. The mercury, in proportion to its degree of volatility, produces tremors, mortifications in the ligaments, madneſs, phrenſy, and delirium. Fevers, phlegmons, impoſthumations, and the jaundice, are the offſpring of the ſulphureous principle; and the cholick, ſtone, gravel, gout, and ſciatica derive their origin from ſalt. What fatal errors in the treatment of diſeaſes, muſt ſuch idle notions of their cauſes, unavoidably produce? The medicines which Paracelſus and his followers employed, were generally metallic preparations, which in ſuch raſh and preſumptuous hands, were doubtleſs, frequently pernicious, and always dangerous. Their common purge in every diſorder was *mercurius*

præci-

præcipitatus, reduced to pills, and made up with the *theriaca* or *mithridate*. About a century after Paracelſus, Van Helmont took the lead in phyſick; a man of ſuch indefatigable induſtry, thar he ſpent fifty years in torturing by every chemical experiment the animal, vegetable, and mineral kingdoms. He was a perſon of learning, and ability, but like his predeceſſor, had the folly of pretending to a univerſal remedy. *(a)* By his writings he defended, enlarged, and promoted, the chemical theory; and as Sylvius de la Boe, and Otho Tachenius ſoon after adopted his ſyſtem, it became almoſt univerſal. All the operations of nature in the world at large, as well as in the animal œconomy, were reduced to the laws of chemiſtry; and

(a) Veteres chemici, quorum interpres eſt Helmontius dixerunt, in cuprum inſitum eſſe genium metallicum, qui vix mole corporea, ſed tantum irradiatione ſanat omnes fere morbos; et Helmontius dixit, hoc fieri ſolo attactu tincturæ cupri ad linguam.

Boerhaave de morb. Nervor. p. 764.

and every phœnomenon was accounted for, on the principles of fermentation, putrefaction, corrosion, effervescence, solution, or mixture. The functions of the body were explained by analogies drawn from chemical experiments. Thus the solution of the aliments in the stomach was ascribed to an acid, because acids were observed to dissolve metals, and other substances of the firmest texture. Muscular motion was accounted for, by an effervescence and explosion in the imaginary rhomboidal receptacles, resembling the tumults raised by the mixture of an acid and an alkali. The generation of animal heat, was imputed to the combination of the acid chyle with a supposed balsam of the blood, because a similar effect is produced by uniting acids with distilled oils. If the acid of the chyle happen to be highly concentrated, and the juices very acrimonious, according to this theory, an ardent fever is excited. The cold fit of an intermittent, was ascribed to the action of

nitre

nitre, ſea ſalt, or ſal ammoniac in the blood, becauſe theſe ſubſtances were found to refrigerate water in a remarkable degree.

FROM this abſurd and groundleſs theory, the practice of the chemical ſect was deduced; of which I ſhall give one memorable and fatal inſtance. In the year 1669 an epedemic fever raged at Leyden, and carried off more than two thirds of the principal inhabitants of that city. The ſymptoms which accompanied it were a diſordered ſtomach, vomitings, anxiety, quotidian or tertian paroxyſms, ſpots, oozing of blood from different parts of the body, dyſenteric ſtools, fœtid urine, great debility, apthæ, and other appearances which indicated a very high degree of putrefaction. But Sylvius de la Boe, who was at that time a Profeſſor in the Univerſity of Leyden, aſcribed the diſtemper to a prevailing acid, and attempted the cure of it by abſorbents and other medicines

medicines of a ſeptic nature; to which injudicious practice we may juſtly impute a conſiderable ſhare of that uncommon fatality which attended the progreſs of this fever. And is it not more than probable, that the preſent practice of giving the *teſtacea* in acute diſtempers hath a dangerous and pernicious tendency? If acidities prevail in the *primæ viæ* they will indeed correct them; but with this inconvenience, that they generally occaſion coſtiveneſs. And if they remain unneutraliſed in the firſt paſſages, they will powerfully promote putrefaction, and by concreting with the mucus of the ſtomach and bowels, prove highly oppreſſive and injurious.

I HAD almoſt omitted to mention a theory of the moſt dangerous tendency, which the chemiſts adopted from Galen, and enriched with many abſurd additions of their own invention. They ſuppoſed the body to be endued with certain *animal*

mal ſpirits, as they were called, generated in a manner ſimilar to that of obtaining brandy from wine by diſtillation. Theſe ſpirits were conſidered as the ſeat of various diſeaſes, particularly of inflammation; and were thought capable of being infected with *ſomething* of a peculiarly deleterious nature. Hence it became a *deſideratum* to expel this unknown enemy out of the ſyſtem; and as it was obſerved that acute diſtempers are ſometimes terminated by a critical ſweat, it was concluded that the moſt powerful ſudorifics were the beſt means of accompliſhing this deſirable end. This gave riſe to the deſtructive and fatal practice, which ſoon became univerſal, of adminiſtering heating remedies in diſeaſes of an inflammatory nature; a practice productive of great devaſtation amongſt the inhabitants of Europe. Sydenham, the Engliſh Hippocrates, was the firſt phyſician who had underſtanding and courage enough, to ſtem the rapid and overwhelming torrent:

rent; and we are now at laſt taught by ſad experience, founded on the deſtruction of numbers of our fellow creatures, that the cooling regimen is alone to be employed in ſuch diſtempers. The ſmall-pox affords us a remarkable example of the oppoſite effects of the two different methods of treatment. And the amazing ſucceſs which hath attended the new mode of inoculation, is a proof, undeniably convincing, of the excellence and ſafety of the one, and of the danger and frequent fatality of the other. So powerful is the action of heating remedies in this diſorder, that a ſingle glaſs of moun tain wine, given even after the eruption is compleated, is ſaid to have produced an additional number of puſtules.

THE ſyſtem of Stahl, which ſucceeded that of the chemiſts, though falſe and abſurd, is not chargeable with any pernicious tendency. As it chiefly relates to the influence of the mind over the body, the doctrine of diseases which it inculcates is simple, and the indications of cure which it furnishes, are few and at least harmless. Thus when the soul in her efforts to relieve the body runs into excess, and excites an immoderate hæmorrhage, *diarrhœa*, or fever, she is to be checked and restrained. On the contrary when she acts negligently or too feebly, she is to be roused and stimulated to an exertion of her powers. In these instances the conclusions of the Stahlians, though deduced from groundless principles, are certainly just, and their practice is supported by experience, the true standard of fitness and propriety in physick.

THE Mechanic Theory, though better supported than the Stahlian, hath a more dangerous influence on the treatment of diseases. Thus, for example, in the management of the small-pox, a physician who is strongly attached to the system of obstruction, and regardless of experience,

perience, might commit the moſt fatal errors. As the diſtemper, according to the mechanical hypotheſis, conſiſts in a certain matter thrown off from the blood, and locked up in the capillaries of the ſkin, where being gradually accumulated it forms puſtules; he would probably attempt either to diſperſe it by repeated purging and venæſection, or to promote its paſſage through the ſmall cutaneous veſſels, by the moſt powerful ſudorifics. The firſt method of cure would occaſion a ſudden ſinking of the pocks; the ſecond would render them putrid, confluent, and malignant. And thus the unfortunate patient would fall a ſacrifice to reaſoning and theory. I mean not by this illuſtration, to charge the mechanic ſect with having adopted ſo dangerous a method of treating the diſeaſe under conſideration. The plan of cure preſcribed by Boerhaave is judicious and ſucceſsful; but it is a deviation from his favourite hypotheſis of obſtruction, and is founded on experience and obſervation. There are however ſome fatal inſtances, in which the mechanical ſyſtematics have regulated their practice by their theory. How many unhappy wretches fell by the lancet, or ſunk under the operation of cathartics, in the ulcerated ſore throat, till the ſagacious Fothergill pointed out the true nature, and right management of that diſeaſe? It is not long ſince crude mercury was conſidered as a *panacea*, and taken univerſally by the healthy as well as the ſick, to prevent obſtructions in the one, and to break down by its gravity thoſe which were already formed in the other. On the ſame principle, the ſpirit and ſalt of hartſhorn were exhibited indiſcriminately in almoſt every ailment; for as they colliquate the blood when taken out of the body, it was not doubted but they would diſſolve that lentor of the fluids which was, and is ſtill by many, regarded as the moſt general cauſe of diſeaſes.

IT

It is evident then that THEORY is absurd and fallacious, always useless, and often in the highest degree pernicious. The annals of medicine afford the most striking proof, that it hath in all ages been the bane and disgrace of the healing art. And as it favours the indolence, flatters the vanity, and gratifies the curiosity of man, ever inquisitive after causes, I fear the passion for it will not be easily suppressed amongst the professors of medicine. The invention of an hypothesis is a work of no difficulty to a lively imagination; and the fiction by its tinsel glitter, never fails to dazzle the ignorant and vulgar. But to watch with close attention the operations of nature, to treasure up a store of useful facts, to learn by accurate observations the diagnostics of diseases, and by unbiassed experience, the true method of cure, requires unwearied labour, assiduity, and patience, at the same time that it admits of no pompous display of wit or knowledge.

The wiſe, however, value not genuine ſcience leſs, for her unaſſuming deportment, and ſimplicity of attire; and the opinion of the ignorant would be unworthy the conſideration of a judicious phyſician, if humanity did not intereſt him in the concerns of ſuch numbers of his fellow creatures, who unhappily fall under that denomination.

ESSAY

ESSAY II.

THE

DOGMATIC;

OR,

ARGUMENTS FOR THE USE

OF

THEORY AND REASONING

IN PHYSIC.

Experientia fallax, judicium difficile.

HIPPOC.

Medicina in philosophia non fundata, res infirma est.

BACON.

ESSAY II.

THE

DOGMATIC;

OR,

RATIONALIST.

THOUGH reaſon is the moſt exalted faculty of man, and the ſource of that high rank which he holds in the univerſe of God, there is a ſet of groveling ſpirits in the world, who vilify the powers of the underſtanding, and with inverted pride, glory in ſinking themſelves to a level with the brute creation. Of this claſs are the EMPIRICS, who have laboured

laboured with infinite pains, to baniſh all theory and reaſoning from the art of medicine. Experience, they affirm, is the ſole guide to ſafe and ſucceſsful practice; and fatal is the temerity of ſuch who deviate from the beaten path, and truſt in any inſtance to the direction of their underſtandings. The proximate cauſe and hidden nature of diſeaſes are beyond our ken, and it is equally abſurd and uſeleſs to attempt their inveſtigation. All that is neceſſary to their cure is plain and obvious, and requires no deep or philoſophical reſearches. We know the ailments to which the human body is incident; we are acquainted alſo with a variety of active remedies; and *uſe* alone hath taught us to adapt the one to the other. Thus argue the empirics; with a ſagacity adequate to the rank of beings, to which by their contempt of reaſon they degrade themſelves. The ſubject however is worthy of an attentive examination.

THERE

THERE are two methods of acquiring experience in the art of medicine; one by reading, the other by practice. The first opens to our view a wide and almost boundless scene of knowledge, presenting us with the lore of all preceding ages: the last is limited and confined, and furnishes a very scanty harvest of instruction. Both are necessary to form the skilful and expert physician; but without the concurring assistance of our judgment and understanding, neither of them will be found of any other avail, than to perplex us with uncertainty, and to lead us into error.

WHOEVER sits down to study the volumes, ancient and modern, which have been written on the subject of medicine, will be amazed at the multiplicity, and confounded with the contrariety of the facts and observations which he meets with. And if he read with no other view than

than to inform himſelf of the experience, and blindly to ſubmit to the direction of his predeceſſors in the healing art, he will either remain in perpetual doubt and ſuſpence, or will treaſure up an indigeſted maſs of contradictory materials, burthenſome to his memory, and unfit for uſe. An undiſtinguiſhing credulity is in no ſcience ſo abſurd and dangerous as in phyſic. Here every fact which is advanced ſhould be examined with accuracy, and admitted with caution. The hiſtories of diſeaſes are frequently the records of falſhood; at leaſt they contain ſuch a mixture of error and truth, as requires the exertion of reaſon, and an extenſive knowledge of the animal œconomy, to ſeparate the one from the other. Still more dubious and uncertain is the therapeutic part of medicine, which hath been ſubject to all the viciſſitudes of faſhion, and regulated by the follies, prejudices, and paſſions of men. How many *panaceas* have been obtruded on the

the world, whoſe miraculous effects have ceaſed the moment they became known? Every author hath his favourite remedy; and what he extols perhaps another may condemn; each pleading in his own behalf the teſtimony of experience. The annals of phyſick abound with inſtances of this kind: thus Hippocrates, Galen, Sydenham, and Boerhaave, with numberleſs other inferior names, are enliſted on the ſide of venæſection; whilſt Eraſiſtratus, Paracelſus, Van Helmont, and the Carteſian ſect, totally baniſh it from the circle of practice. A ſimilar fate hath attended the other means of evacuation; and purgatives and emetics, at different times, have been ſtrongly recommended, or ignominiouſly proſcribed. Antimony was formerly conſidered as a poiſon, and its uſe was forbidden by a publick edict at Rome; whereas now it is employed under various forms, and conſtitutes one of the moſt valuable articles of the *materia*

teria medica. The Peruvian Bark ſoon after its introduction into Europe, met with the moſt powerful oppoſition. Numberleſs miſchiefs were aſcribed to its operation, and caſes recited wherein its effects were ſaid to be obviouſly pernicious. Even thoſe who thought the moſt favourably of it, regarded it as a dangerous though efficacious medicine, and never adminiſtered it, but with caution and reſerve. At preſent it is given in the largeſt doſes, and in ſuch a variety of diſorders, that it is become an almoſt univerſal remedy. Opium, Steel, and Mercury, have alſo undergone their ſeveral revolutions, and the moſt contradictory teſtimonies may be collected concerning their nature and effects. Theſe few inſtances (for many more might be adduced) ſufficiently prove the abſurdity of blindly adopting the experience of *others*; and it will be found on examination that *our own*, without the aſſiſtance of theory and reaſoning, is

no

no leſs expoſed to uncertainty and error. The diſeaſes to which the human body is obnoxious are ſo various, and frequently ſo complicated with each other, that it requires the cleareſt judgment to diſtinguiſh them with accuracy, and the niceſt ſkill to treat them with propriety. Their ſymptoms are to be weighed with attention ſeparately as well as collectively; the temperament, age, and ſex of the patient are to be conſidered; and the remote, and occaſional cauſes of ſickneſs to which he may have been expoſed, are to be examined into, before any concluſion can be drawn concerning the *genus* of the ailment, or the indications of cure. In the application of remedies, regard is to be had to the nature, internal ſource and period of the diſtemper, and to the peculiar habit or idioſyncraſy of the ſick perſon. But this implies the exerciſe of reaſon, and beſides experience requires a knowledge of the ſtructure and functions of the animal frame, of the changes pro-

duced

duced in it by diſeaſe, and of the powers and qualities of medicines: all which the empiric rejects as viſionary and uſeleſs. "In a watch every one obſerves when the finger deviates, but the artiſt alone, who is acquainted with the exquiſite ſtructure of the machine, can correct and amend its movements." A conſtant and diligent attendance on the ſick, may inſtruct us in the external face of diſeaſes, and enable us with ſome degree of certainty to prognoſticate their iſſue. But without theory and an exertion of our rational faculties, it will never furniſh any other than the mere fortuitous means of relieving them. The ſavage Indian, by his accurate obſervation of natural ſigns, can frequently foretel thoſe tremendous ſtorms to which America, at certain ſeaſons, is expoſed: But of what avail would this have been in preventing the impending ruin, if philoſophy had not accompliſhed what was impoſſible to rude experience? To the ingenious Franklin our

our colonies owe the warmeſt gratitude, who by inveſtigating the nature and cauſes of thunder and lightning, hath pointed out the method of warding off their deſtructive effects. How bind and dangerous would be all attempts to cure the diſorders of the eye, without a knowledge of its ſtructure, and an acquaintance with the theory of viſion? And yet the empiric is profeſſedly ignorant of both. Suppoſe him to be conſulted by a patient labouring under the *gutta ſerena*: no external defect appears, no pain is complained of, and the health of the body in every other reſpect is perhaps unimpaired. By what ſigns will he be able to determine the ſeat of the diſeaſe; or upon what principles will he proceed in the treatment of it? Confuſion, uncertainty, and danger muſt neceſſarily attend his random practice. By the laws of the animal œconomy, there ſubſiſts a certain ſympathy between different parts of the body; by which the diſordered ſtate of one organ impairs the functions of another. The head and ſtomach, for inſtance, have an almoſt univerſal conſent with the reſt of the ſyſtem, and of conſequence are ſubject to various and ſometimes oppoſite cauſes of indiſpoſition, each indicating a different and peculiar method of cure. Thus watching, flatulency, indigeſtion, the gout, rheumatiſm, or inflammation, may produce the head-ach; and ſickneſs or vomiting may ariſe from ſurfeiting, from a load of mucus, from putrid bile, from an affection of the kidneys, and, from many other ſources. In all theſe caſes the empiric, if he act conſiſtently with his principles, will attend only to the leading ſymptom, and will indiſcriminately apply his ſtomachic cordial, or cephalic plaiſter, without any regard to the origin or nature of the malady.

MAY we not therefore juſtly conclude, that mere experience, whether derived from

from books, or acquired by perſonal obſervation, is inſufficient of itſelf to qualify us for judicious and ſucceſsful practice. "I look upon a good Phyſician," ſays the amiable Mr. Boyle, "not properly as a ſervant to nature, but as a counſellor and friendly aſſiſtant, who in his patients body furthers every thing which he judges to be conducive to the welfare and recovery of it." To this end a knowledge of the animal œconomy, of the influence of external cauſes on the human frame, of the ſtate of health, and the changes induced by diſeaſe, is abſolutely neceſſary. And this is the foundation on which the Rationaliſt erects the ſuperſtructure of medicine. He explores the writings of the ancients and moderns, he attends diligently to nature in her operations, he ſelects and arranges facts, and deduces general concluſions, and thus forms a conſiſtent, rational, and uſeful theory, on which his practice is built. (a) He neither indulges a warm and creative imagination, nor yet confines himself within the limits of one narrow hypothesis, well knowing the absurdity of either extreme. With the Stahlians he believes that the soul, or nature, as it is now called, frequently exerts herself in the cure of diseases, or in expelling from the body whatever is offensive and hurtful. Thus a *crapula* occasions a *diarrhœa*, and a crumb of bread in the wind-pipe excites a fit of coughing. But he is aware likewise, that the efforts of nature in such cases may be too powerful; that a salutary *diarrhœa* may terminate in a dysentery, and a fit of coughing in universal convulsions. He adopts also, with restric-

(a) ALTHOUGH the arguing from experiments and observations by induction, be no demonstration of general conclusions, yet it is the best way of arguing which the nature of things admits of; and may be looked upon as so much the stronger, by how much the induction is more general.

NEWTON.

reſtrictions, the mechanical and chemical hypotheſes, and admits that obſtruction is often a cauſe of diſeaſe, and that many changes in the body are reducible to chemical and mechanical principles, of which he deems inflammation and acrimony to be ſufficient proofs. But he is not wedded to ſyſtems, nor anxiouſly bent upon explaining every phœnomenon which occurs in the animal frame. He diligently avails himſelf indeed of all the aſſiſtances with which philoſophy furniſhes the healing art; but ſenſible of its imperfection, he ingenuouſly acknowledges that in diſeaſes there are numberleſs anomalous ſymptoms, that the operation of medicines is often irregular and uncertain, and that even in the healthy body there are many appearances, which are inexplicable to the wiſeſt and moſt experienced of the faculty. But where his theory is deficient, his practice is proportionably more cautious and reſerved. If experience fails him, he calls in analogy to his aid; *(a)* and judges it better to purſue a doubtful path, than to ſtand ſtill in uncertainty and ſuſpenſe. In the moſt intricate caſes, however, he is not totally without a clue: Reaſon and philoſophy are his guides; and under ſuch direction, there is at leaſt a probability that he will not miſtake his courſe. And by thus treading occaſionally in unbeaten tracks, he enlarges the boundaries of ſcience in general, and adds new diſcoveries to the art of medicine. In a word, the Rationaliſt has every advantage which the Empiric can boaſt, from reading, obſervation, and practice, accompanied with ſuperior knowledge, underſtanding, and judgment.

(a) EJUS (analogiæ) hæc vis eſt, ut id quod dubium eſt, ad aliquod ſimile de quo non quæritur, referat; ut incerta certis probet.

Quint. Inſt. Orat l. 1. c. 6.

ESSAY

ESSAY III.

EXPERIMENTS AND OBSERVATIONS ON ASTRINGENTS AND BITTERS.

Nata est ars ab experimento.

QUINTILIAN.

E S S A Y III.

EXPERIMENTS AND OBSERVATIONS ON ASTRINGENTS AND BITTERS.

EXPERIMENT I.

AN ounce of PERUVIAN BARK, coarſely powdered, was divided into two equal parts, one of which was infuſed forty eight hours, in ſix ounces of cold ſpring water; the other was boiled over a ſlow fire forty minutes, in nine ounces of water, till about a third part of the water was evaporated. The infuſion and decoction were each filtered through linen rags doubled, and of equal fineneſs.

FOUR

FOUR grains of *ſal martis* were diſſolved in an ounce of ſpring water, and one drachm of this ſolution was added to equal quantities (viz. half an ounce) of the turbid decoction and infuſion. Each aſſumed a deep purple colour, ſcarce perceptibly different in degree, though I thought the infuſion, after ſtanding a while, acquired rather a more duſky purple than the decoction. The infuſion had a deeper tinge, and more of the taſte and ſmell of the bark in ſubſtance than the decoction: Its taſte indeed exactly reſembled the bark, after it has been broken down, and chewed for ſome time in the mouth.

EXPERIMENT II.

EQUAL quantities of each *reſiduum* were boiled over a ſlow fire in three ounces of ſpring water, for the ſpace of twenty minutes. The decoctions were equally turbid, exactly ſimilar in taſte,

and

and on the addition of the chalybeate ſolution, in the proportion of one drachm to half an ounce, they aſſumed preciſely the ſame colour, viz. a duſky brown like chocolate. but inclining ſomewhat to purple.

EXPERIMENT III.

Five drachms of each *reſiduum* were infuſed for the ſpace of forty hours, in an ounce and an half of Jamaica Rum, which was ſufficiently pure, and unimpregnated with any aſtringent matter from the caſk. The tinctures were exactly alike in taſte and colour; and on the addition of one drachm of the chalybeate ſolution, they were inſtantly changed from a deep red to a dark and dirty brown, which was preciſely the ſame in both tinctures.

EXPE-

EXPERIMENT IV.

To half an ounce of powdered bark was added an ounce of cold ſpring water. The mixture was well triturated in a marble mortar, after which it was ſuffered to remain at reſt till the groſs powder ſubſided. The clear liquor was then carefully poured off, and freſh water to the quantity of half an ounce was added; the trituration was renewed, and afterwards part of the *menſtruum* poured off again as before. This method was purſued for the ſpace of thirty four hours, in which time ſix ounces of water were combined with the bark. The mixture was then infuſed fourteen hours, without heat, and ſtrained off. This infuſion was found to have the ſmell and taſte of the bark, in a conſiderably greater degree than either the decoction, or the infuſion without trituration, [Exper. I.] and it aſſumed a much blacker colour,

lour, on mixing with it one drachm of the chalybeate ſolution, than either of the two former preparations.

EXPERIMENT V.

It was attempted to determine the comparative ſtrength, or rather aſtringency, of five preparations of the bark, viz. the extract, decoction, cold infuſion, tincture, and triturated infuſion.

Ten grains of the extract carefully made, and as free from *empyreuma* as this officinal preparation is generally found to be, were mixed with an ounce of hot water. But ſo imperfect was the ſolution, or to ſpeak more properly the ſuſpenſion of the bark, that in a few minutes a large powder was depoſited at the bottom of the glaſs. This however was ſhaken up, and one drachm of the chalybeate ſolution was added to the mixture. The ſame quantity was added

to

to half an ounce of the decoction, infusion, tincture of the London Dispensatory, and triturated infusion. The last assumed by far the deepest black, the extract approached nearest to it, and the tincture appeared to be the least tinged. The decoction and infusion were precisely alike in colour.

EXPERIMENT VI.

THE *residuum* of the triturated infusion, [Exper. IV.] was boiled over a slow fire in three ounces of water, for the space of twenty minutes. The decoction when cold was strained off. It was of a paler colour than the decoctions mentioned in Exper. II. although there was a portion of powdered bark suspended in it, which, by the trituration, had been rendered fine enough to pass through the filter. This powder on standing subsided to the bottom of the vessel, and left the decoction

coction much more limpid than it was before.

To equal quantities of this and of the two decoctions mentioned above, one drachm of the chalybeate solution was added. The black tinge was manifestly weakest in this decoction, though the difference was not so great as might have been expected from the diversity in their sensible qualities of taste and smell; owing perhaps to the fine powder of the bark which floated in it, and retained some degree of its original astringency.

EXPERIMENT VII.

Equal quantities of the simple and of the triturated infusion, were boiled for the space of seven minutes over a quick fire. Both lost their transparency when cool; but the latter assumed a much more turbid appearance than the former,

former, exceeding even that of the decoction from fresh bark [Exper. I.] and after standing twenty four hours, it deposited a very copious sediment.

EXPERIMENT VIII.

HALF an ounce of powdered bark was infused forty eight hours, in five ounces of spring water, and one ounce of white wine vinegar. The mixture was placed near a warm fire, and at certain intervals was smartly shaken. It was then filtered through a linen rag doubled. The taste of the vinegar was in a good measure covered, though the smell was not; but the *menstruum* was not so fully impregnated with the flavour of the bark as the infusion. [Exper. I.] One drachm of the chalybeate solution was added to half an ounce of this acid infusion; at first no change of colour took place, but in a few hours a slight black tinge appeared.

EXPE-

EXPERIMENT IX.

HALF an ounce of powdered bark was well triturated, in the manner described in exper. IV. with ſix ounces of warm water; after which the mixture was poured into a bottle, placed near the fire, and frequently ſhaken. This proceſs laſted forty eight hours. The infuſion, when ſtrained off, was found to be more perfectly impregnated with the bark, than the triturated infuſion with cold water [Exper. IV.] as appeared by comparing their colour, taſte, and ſmell, and by the deeper black which it inſtantly aſſumed on the mixture of one drachm of the ſolution of *ſal martis*.

EXPERIMENT X.

HALF an ounce of powdered bark, and two drachms of ſtone quick lime, warm from the kiln, were rubbed together until they were thoroughly united; then ſix ounces of ſpring water were gradually poured on, the powder and water were well incorporated by triture, and the mixture was ſet by to infuſe for twelve hours. Two ounces of it were then filtered through a double linen cloth: the remainder ſtood thirty ſix hours longer, and was often agitated; after which it was ſtrained off. The ſmell of the bark was almoſt entirely covered in both the infuſions, which were ſtrongly impregnated with the lime, and had an extremely diſagreeable flavour. The firſt was of a pale colour, and poſſeſſed but a ſlight degree of bitterneſs; the latter had a deeper tinge, and was equally bitter and nauſeous. Neither of them ſtruck a black colour with the chalybeate ſolution, which as ſoon as it was added occaſioned the ſeparation of a yellow ſediment, which in a few hours ſubſided to the bottom of the glaſs. Compared with the triturated infuſion

[Exper.

[Exper. IV.] theſe preparations appeared to be much weaker both in colour and taſte. The *reſiduum* did not ſenſibly efferveſce with oil of vitriol.

EXPERIMENT XI.

The decoction and infuſion, were found to be impaired in ſtrength after ſtanding ſix or ſeven days; although it was the winter ſeaſon, and the weather was ſeverely cold. The infuſion became paler coloured, and at the ſame time depoſited a ſlimy ſediment. The decoction at the end of ſeven days, aſſumed an almoſt milky hue, and ſtruck but a faint black with the chalybeate ſolution. The ſimple infuſion alſo had loſt much of its aſtringency; but the two triturated infuſions were very little altered in that reſpect.

EXPERIMENT XII.

To determine the time requiſite for

obtaining a ſufficiently ſtrong impregnation of the Peruvian bark in cold water; four infuſions were prepared, by macerating equal quantities (two drachms) of the fine powder of the *cortex*, in four ounces of rain water. *(a)* After two hours infuſion, the firſt was filtered; the ſecond after ſeven hours; the third after nineteen hours; and the fourth after forty eight hours. The ſecond infuſion, which had been prepared by ſeven hours maceration, appeared by its taſte, ſmell, colour, and by the hue which it aſſumed on dropping into it a ſaturated ſolution of green vitriol, to be conſiderably more impregnated with the bark than the firſt, and to be equal in ſtrength to the other two preparations. This experiment demonſtrates that the *cortex* yields its virtues,

(a) THE foregoing infuſions of the bark would have been ſtronger, had they been made with the fine powder of the cortex; and they would have ſtruck a deeper black with green vitriol, had a leſs quantity of the chalybeate been employed.

tues, in a ſhort time, to cold water, and that it is unneceſſary to continue the infuſion longer than ſeven or eight hours.

Physicians in general agree, that the peruvian bark is moſt powerful in its effects when taken in ſubſtance. But as the ſtomach is frequently unable to bear it, and as many patients have an almoſt invincible averſion to it in that form, it is of importance to determine in what preparations the virtues of this valuable drug are leaſt impaired, and whether it may not be adminiſtered under a form that is elegant, palatable, and at the ſame time ſufficiently efficacious. The decoction of the bark hath always appeared to me, to be an injudicious preparation: for though the *cortex* is not a ſubſtance of much volatility, *(a)* yet

F 3 there

(a) Astringency is perhaps not ſo fixed a quality in vegetables, as is commonly ſuppoſed; for I am well informed

there is a certain *aroma* accompanying it, which the heat of boiling water cannot fail to diſſipate; *(a)* and conſequently the medicine is deprived of one of its component parts, in which probably ſome ſhare of its virtues reſides. The bark likewiſe undergoes a decompoſition by boiling; the reſin is ſeparated from the gum, and remains ſuſpended in the watery *menſtruum*. This renders its appearance inelegant, its taſte nauſeous, and, I ſhould apprehend, muſt conſiderably

informed that artichoke ſtalks, by being gently dried in an oven, loſe their property of ſtriking a black colour with chalybeates.

(a) THE vapour which exhales in the firſt coction, being caught in proper veſſels, condenſes into a limpid liquor which ſmells ſtrongly of the bark.

Lewis's Mat. Med. p. 431.

GENUINUS cortex, ſapore ſatis grato, et aromatice-amaro eſt; odorem ſpirat peculiari modo mucidum, attamen ſuavem, gratum, et *aromaticum*; atque huic ſenſui, in corticis ſinceritate deprehendenda, præ cæteris omnibus credere ſoleo.

Morton. lib. 1. p. 66.

ably diminiſh its efficacy. For as the virtues of the bark are ſtrongeſt in its native ſtate, they depend in all probability on its compoſition as a *mixt*; and muſt of courſe be impaired by the diſuniting of its conſtituent principles. Intermittents have been cured by oak bark and gentian combined, when neither aſtringents nor bitters ſeparately, had any effect. By the firſt, ſecond, and third experiments it appears, that the *cortex* yields its virtues at leaſt as perfectly to cold as to boiling water. And the ſimple infuſion hath certainly many advantages over the decoction. It is a much more agreeable and elegant preparation, and the principles of the bark remain perfectly unaltered in it, retaining the ſame proportions to each other as in the ſubſtance of the drug itſelf. Nature hath ſo accurately combined, and blended together the gummy and reſinous parts of the *cortex*, that by their union they become ſoluble in *menſtrua*, with which when ſeparated they refuſe to unite. Thus they reciprocally promote the ſolution of each other in water and ardent ſpirits; and both the tincture and infuſion are found by experiment, to be ſtrongly impregnated with theſe two conſtituent principles of the bark. The tincture is without doubt an elegant and palatable medicine; but it is liable to this objection, which indeed holds equally true againſt ſpirituous tinctures in general, that a ſufficient doſe of the medicine cannot be given, on account of the heating nature of its vehicle. This preparation however, might be rendered much ſtronger, if a larger proportion of bark, than is preſcribed by the college of phyſicians, were to be employed.

EXPERIMENT XIII.

EQUAL quantities, viz. ſix ounces by meaſure of two tinctures of the bark, the one made after the *formula* of the London Diſpen-

Diſpenſatory, the other with double the uſual quantity of bark, were weighed with great exactneſs, in a nice pair of ſcales; and the latter was found to be eighteen grains heavier than the former, and to exceed in gravity the ſimple proof ſpirit thirty ſeven grains. The ſtronger tincture had alſo a conſiderably deeper hue, and when mixed with water became much more turbid.

In nervous fevers, hyſterical diſorders, and other low caſes where it is neceſſary to join cordials to the bark, an infuſion of it in red port wine may be preſcribed with advantage. Under this form the famous empiric Talbot uſed to adminiſter the *cortex* in the paroxyſms of intermittents; and ſo ſucceſsful was his practice, that Louis XIV. was induced to purchaſe at a large price the ſecret of his ſpecific. Orange peel is an uſeful ingredient in preparations of the bark; it gives a grateful warmth to the infuſion, and

and adds, I think, conſiderably to its efficacy. The following *formula* is agreeable to the taſte, and well adapted to a weak and delicate ſtomach.

℞ *Pulv. cort. peruv.* ℥j. *cort. aurant.* ℥ſs. *aq. cinnamom. ten.* ℔j. *aq. cinnamom. ſp.* ℥ij. *m. et infunde ſine calore per horas octo, vel duodecim, deinde filtra.*

The uſe of trituration in promoting the powers of ſolution is evident from experiments IV. VI. and VII; and would have been ſtill more ſo, if a proper apparatus had been employed. The Count de la Garaye, a French nobleman, who is diſtinguiſhed for his aſſiduity in applying the different branches of philoſophy to the improvement of medicine, hath deſcribed a very convenient machine, and pointed out an admirable proceſs for obtaining from vegetables, by triture with water, the matters in which their virtues chiefly reſide.

reſide. The contrivance is extremely ſimple, conſiſting only of a veſſel to which a churning ſtaff is fitted, which by means of a cord and a wheel, is perpetually whirled with a rotatory motion. By this conſtant agitation the moſt accurate diffuſion is produced, and different portions of the *menſtruum* are in quick ſucceſſion applied to every particle of the ſolvend.

FROM the 5th. experiment no certain concluſions can be deduced; except that the extract is a much weaker preparation than is commonly ſuppoſed. It is liable to all the objections which have been advanced againſt the decoction, with this additional one, that it is hardly poſſible to make it according to the proceſs of the London Diſpenſatory, without giving it ſome degree of *empyreuma*. The extract employed in my experiment, was prepared by a very diligent and careful apothecary, yet a conſiderable portion of it

preſently

prefently fubfided in a powdery form to the bottom of the glafs, which on examination appeared to be the burnt parts of the bark. How little then is this officinal medicine to be depended upon, when we confider the careleffnefs and inaccuracy of many of our druggifts, and apothecaries. (a)

IT

(a) It were to be wifhed, that the college of phyficians would direct all extracts to be made, by means of a water bath. The following fimple contrivance will fully, commodioufly, and with very little trouble to the operator, anfwer this purpofe. Let a pan be made of fuitable dimenfions, with a large circular hole in the cover of it, adapted to receive a china, or glafs bafon, and with a curved pipe, two inches high, and half an inch in diameter, on one fide: the cover fhould be clofely cemented to the pan. Fill the veffel with a fufficient quantity of water; then place the bafon in the cavity defigned to receive it, and lute it well to the cover. The pan may now be fet over a kitchen fire, and the liquor intended for evaporation poured into the china bafon. From the clofenefs of the veffel, the heat which the water acquires will exceed the common boiling point; and the evaporation will be proportionably expedited, without the leaft danger of producing an *empyreuma*. The pipe will ferve the double purpofe of conveying

It is the practice of the moſt eminent phyſicians, to join acids with the bark in the cure of putrid diſeaſes; and Sir John Pringle hath obſerved, that in bilious fevers the *cortex* anſwered beſt in Rheniſh wine, after ſtanding a night in infuſion. (a) This ſuggeſted to me the 8th. experiment, and I flattered myſelf that by macerating the bark in a mixture of vinegar and water, theſe two antiſeptic medicines would be more accurately combined, and that perhaps the acid might promote the diſſolvent power of the aqueous *menſtruum*. In the latter expectation it appears that I was diſappointed; and whether the former was better founded muſt be left to abler judges to determine. (b)

THAT

veying a freſh ſupply of water into the pan, when it is wanted, and of carrying off ſome part of the ſteam. If a greater degree of heat be required, the pipe may be cloſed with a cork.

(a) Diſeaſes of the Army, Edit. 4. p. 213.

(b) Vide Experiments XIX. XXVI.

THAT moderate heat promotes and aſſiſts the action of water, as a *menſtruum*, on the bark, is evident from experiment the IX; and it would be of advantage to determine what degree of heat this drug will admit of, without ſuffering a decompoſition. It ſhould, however, be remarked, that this infuſion though ſtronger, had neither ſo agreeable a flavour, nor was ſo ſenſibly impregnated with the *aroma* of the bark, as the two made with cold water.

IN an eſſay on the DISSOLVENT POWER OF QUICK LIME, a very ingenious chemiſt hath obſerved, that all reſinous bodies become ſoluble in water, when the coheſion of their particles is deſtroyed by withdrawing the fixed air which they contain. This method of ſolution he endeavours to apply to many valuable purpoſes in medicine; and hath deſcribed ſeveral uſeful and curious proceſſes, for obtaining ſtrong and elegant tinctures of the

the moſt active drugs by means of quick-lime. The firſt part of the 10th experiment, *mutatis mutandis*, was borrowed from him; and it was hoped that an efficacious and palatable infuſion, might with tolerable expedition be made, by the proceſs which he has laid down. But the ſucceſs of my experiment was not anſwerable to the plauſibility and ingenuity of the theory, which induced me to attempt it. The infuſion after ſtanding twelve hours, the time preſcribed by Dr. Macbride, was but weakly impregnated with the bark: and when the maceration had been continued forty eight hours, it by no means equalled in ſtrength the preparation deſcribed. Exper. IV. It appears therefore that quick-lime, whatever its effect may be upon other medicines, neither quickens nor increaſes the ſolubility of bark in water: and it communicates to the infuſion a taſte which is intolerably nauſeous and diſagreeable. That the chalybeate ſo-

lution

lution ſhould produce no change in the colour of theſe preparations, is agreeable to the laws of elective attraction. For the acid of the vitriol, having a ſtronger affinity with abſorbent earths than with metallic ſubſtances, forſakes the iron with which it was combined, and unites itſelf to the quick lime. Hence aroſe the yellow, ochery ſediment taken notice of in the experiment. As the *reſiduum* after filtration did not effervefce with oil of vitriol, it is evident that quick lime is not endued with the power of abſtracting from bark, the fixed air which it contains.

Experiment XI. furniſhes no other inference than this obvious one, that the decoction and infuſion of the bark are calculated only for immediate uſe. The *cortex* is a ſubſtance of a very fermentable nature, as appears from the experiments of Dr. Macbride; and when its active parts are diffuſed in water, and ſeparated from

from ſuch as are merely ligneous and inert, it is not to be wondered at that it undergoes thoſe changes, to which all vegetables, when favourably circumſtanced, are liable.

As it is to be feared that decoctions of the bark, from the facility with which they are prepared, will ſtill continue in uſe, it may be neceſſary to ſuggeſt, that they ſhould be poured upon the filter as ſoon as they are taken from the fire. Whilſt the water is hot, the reſinous part of the *cortex* will continue diſſolved in it, and will readily paſs through a coarſe ſtrainer; but if the *menſtruum* be ſuffered to cool, it will ſeparate, concrete together, and a conſiderable portion of it will remain in the filter: and thus the efficacy of the medicine will be greatly diminiſhed.

SECTION II.

IT appears from the preceding ſection, that the PERUVIAN BARK yields its virtues as perfectly to cold as to boiling water; and that the ſimple infuſion in point of elegance and efficacy, is preferable to the decoction. But the latter preparation hath this advantage, that it is made with great expedition: For it is a fundamental principle in chemiſtry, that heat quickens the action of almoſt every *menſtruum*. To avail myſelf therefore of this aſſiſtance without decompoſing the bark, I made the following experiment, in the iſſue of which it will appear that I was diſappointed.

EXPE-

EXPERIMENT XIV.

A GLASS phial lightly ſtopped, containing two drachms of powdered bark, well incorporated with three ounces of ſpring water, was placed in a half pint cup of cold water. The cup was ſet in a pan of boiling water, and kept in the boiling heat for the ſpace of an hour and half. The phial was then taken out of the veſſel, and the heat of it meaſured by Sir Iſaac Newton's thermometer, when it was found to be about eight degrees below the boiling point, which is nearly equal to forty degrees in Farenheit's ſcale. The infuſion whilſt hot was clear, and of a deep red, but when cold, it aſſumed a brown colour, and had a turbid appearance.

SEVERAL other experiments were tried, in order to determine what degree of heat the bark will bear without decompoſition; but I was unable to hit upon the precise point. And when I considered that if it could be ascertained, few apothecaries in extemporaneous prescriptions would pay an exact attention to it, I dropt all further attempts towards the discovery of it. But the following experiment, which I have made since the first edition of these Essays, obviates the necessity of using heat, and points out a method of making, with sufficient ease and expedition, a saturated infusion of the bark.

EXPERIMENT XV.

Two drachms of the *cortex*, finely powdered, were diligently triturated, fifteen minutes, in a marble mortar, with four ounces of rain water; and afterwards macerated without heat, three quarters of an hour. The infusion was then filtered through paper, and appeared by all the tests used in the preceding expe-

experiments, to be conſiderably ſtronger than another preparation, which had been macerated twenty four hours. Three ounces of it, by meaſure, weighed a grain and half more than the infuſion, prepared, according to the ſame proportions, without attrition.

A SIMILAR preparation was made by triturating the *cortex* ten minutes only, and then filtering without digeſtion. But the *menſtruum* was by this method, leſs impregnated with the bark, as its taſte, colour, ſpecific gravity, and the diminiſhed effect of the chalybeate ſolution, clearly evinced. The elegance, and ſtrength of this preparation is increaſed, by the addition of a ſmall quantity of French brandy, during the triture.

EXPERIMENT XVI.

IT is evident from the 7th experiment, that a conſiderable quantity of the resin of the bark is soluble in cold water; but I was desirous of trying whether the whole of it might not be dissolved by repeated affusions of the same *menstruum*. For this purpose I macerated half an ounce of powdered bark, for the space of three days, in six ounces of spring water. The *menstruum* was then decanted off, and fresh water added in the same quantity as before. This affusion was repeated at equal intervals thirty times, till the water was insipid, colourless, and unalterable by the addition of green vitriol. The *residuum* also, when chewed in the mouth, had no sensible bitterness or astringency. Two drachms of this *residuum*, carefully dried by a very gentle heat, were infused in an ounce of rectified spirit of wine; and in two days a tincture was produced of an orange colour, and bitter taste.

EXPERIMENT XVII.

Half an ounce of powdered bark loosely

loofely tied up in a linen rag, was boiled over a quick fire twenty five times, in fo many different pints of fpring water. Each coction was continued twenty minutes, and repeated till the *menftruum* received no fenfible impregnation from the bark. After the twenty fifth boiling, it was perfectly taftelefs, ftruck no black with *fal martis*, and the powder when chewed in the mouth was equally infipid with the liquor. Two drachms of the *refiduum*, cautioufly dried, were digefted forty eight hours, in an ounce of *fp. vin. rectificat*. The fpirits acquired a deeper colour, and were more ftrongly impregnated with the bitternefs of the *cortex*, than in the preceding experiment. But neither this, nor the former tincture, ftruck a black with green vitriol, owing perhaps to the infolubility of that metallic falt in rectified fpirit of wine.

EXPERIMENT XVIII.

A DRACHM of powdered bark was digested without heat forty eight hours, in two ounces of rectified ſpirit of wine. The clear tincture was then poured off, and freſh ſpirit, in the ſame quantity as before, was added to the *reſiduum*. The digeſtion was thus repeated ſix times, until the *menſtruum* acquired neither taſte nor colour from the bark. The powder was then carefully dried, and afterwards ſucceſſively macerated, without heat, in two ſeveral portions of ſpring water; to each of which it communicated the property of ſtriking a purple colour with green vitriol. Both theſe infuſions were inſipid; ſo that rectified ſpirit ſeems to have the power of extracting all the bitterneſs of the *cortex*, though not all its aſtringency. Is not this fact repugnant to what Dr. Lewis hath obſerved of this drug, " that its aſtrin-

aſtringency reſides wholly in its reſin, which does not appear to be in any degree ſoluble in watery liquors?"*(a)* The ſame ingenious writer is likewiſe miſtaken, when he aſſerts that the reſin of the bark melts out in the firſt boilings, and that the ſubſequent decoctions are tranſparent and bitter, without the leaſt turbidneſs or aſtringency.*(b)* For in making the 17th experiment, I found the decoction after the twentieth boiling, ſtruck a purple colour with *ſal martis.* The three laſt trials furniſh a ſtriking proof of the ſlow and difficult ſolubility of the bark. Fuller ſays with ſome degree of admiration, *Cum olim experimenti cauſa ejuſdem (corticis) pulverem ſæpius decoxiſſem, non eo uſque vires ejus exhaurire valui, quin vel octavum decoctum adhuc amaricaret.* *(c)* If his patience had permitted

(a) Neumann's Chem. by Lewis, p. 339. Note (x)

(b) Ibid.

(c) Fuller. Pharm. Extemp. p. 5.

mitted him to extend his experiment, what would have been his ſurpriſe to find, that even twenty five coctions, and thirty cold macerations, are inſufficient to exhauſt the virtues of the *cinchona?* An ingenious friend of mine informs me, that he reduced the bark, by extraction and decoction, to an inſipid powder, which was given in the doſe of two drachms, to a patient labouring under a quotidian fever, an hour or two before the acceſſion of the paroxyſm. It mitigated the fits by degrees, changed the quotidian into a tertian, and then entirely removed it.

EXPERIMENT XIX.

IN order to determine with more accuracy the relation which different *menſtrua* bear to the bark, I digeſted a drachm of the *cortex*, weighed with great exactneſs in equal quantities, viz. three ounces of each of the following liquors. 1. ſpirit of of wine rectified. 2. French brandy. 3. Rhenish wine. 4. cold water. 5. cold water with the addition of a drachm and half of white wine vinegar. After seven days infusion, the clear part of each *menstruum* was carefully poured off, and the *residuum* evaporated to dryness. The weight which the bark lost by digestion is expressed in the following table, which shews the comparative powers of solution of the several liquors mentioned above.

Cort. Peruv. ʒj. infused seven days in

		Grains.
Sp. vin. rectificat.	lost	6
Sp. vin. gallic.	—	$8\frac{1}{4}$
Rhenish wine	—	9
Water	—	8
Water and vinegar	—	8

RHENISH wine, from this experiment, appears to be the most active *menstruum* for the bark. Whether it owes any part of its superior solvent power to the acid with

with which it is replete, cannot with certainty be determined; but I am inclined to think it doth not, becaufe the folution of the *cortex* is not in the leaft promoted by the addition of vinegar to water. Dr. Lewis fays, that proof fpirit extracts lefs from bark than rectified fpirit; (a) but from the preceding trial, which was made with all poffible exactnefs, it is evident he is miftaken. This experiment likewife affords the moft fatisfactory proof, that cold water is a powerful *menftruum* for the *cinchona*. It is confiderably more active than rectified fpirit of wine, and is very little inferior to brandy. Perhaps the *refiduum* of the watery infufion would have weighed lefs, if the maceration had been continued only two days: for water, after extracting from bark all that it is capable of diffolving, precipitates fome part of it again.

EXPE-

(a) Mat. Medica. p. 432.

EXPERIMENT XX.

Two drachms of gentian root were macerated forty eight hours, in three ounces of cold ſpring water: the ſame quantity was boiled over a quick fire in four ounces of water, till a fourth part was conſumed. The infuſion had a more intenſely bitter, and at the ſame time a much leſs diſagreeable taſte than the decoction, which was mucilaginous, and highly nauſeous. Six grains of *ſal martis* were added to each; but neither of them changed colour. The ſame experiment was repeated with Aleppo galls. The decoction manifeſted more roughneſs and aſtringency to the taſte, than the infuſion, but did not ſtrike ſo black a colour with green vitriol. Dr. Lewis informs us, that by ſteeping the *carduus benedictus* for a few hours in cold water, a very agreeable bitter is procured; but if heat be employed, the more ungrateful parts of the plant

plant are taken up, and the infusion becomes so nauseous as to provoke vomiting. If sena be infused in cold, or for a little time in warm water, the liquor will purge far more mildly than an infusion made in hot water for a longer time, though both infusions be reduced to the same degree of strength, by a suitable evaporation. *(a)* Camomile flowers, as I have long experienced, have their bitterness very perfectly extracted by cold maceration; and in this way they they are much more grateful, than when infused in boiling water. An ounce of flowers, and half an ounce of orange peel, macerated in three pints of water for twenty four hours, make a light, cheap, and agreeable stomachic medicine. Green and bohea tea yield a finer flavour to a cold than hot infusion, and they strike as deep a black by the former, as by the latter method of preparation. Oak bark, it

(a) Vide Neumann's Chem. p. 267.

it is well known, is always ſteeped in cold water for the purpoſe of tanning: and I ſuppoſe the artiſts in that branch of trade, find that the application of heat is not neceſſary to extract its aſtringency. May we not therefore juſtly conclude from the preceding experiments and obſervations, that cold water is a more univerſal and powerful *menſtruum*, than hath hitherto been apprehended; and that its uſe in pharmacy is at preſent too much overlooked and neglected.

THE reſult of the 8th experiment was ſo contrary to my expectations, that I determined to make further trials of the effects of acids, in deſtroying that property in certain vegetable ſubſtances, by which they ſtrike a black colour with chalybeates, which hath been long regarded as an indubitable teſt of aſtringency.

EXPE-

EXPERIMENT XXI.

An ounce of the infuſion of camomile flowers was divided into two equal portions; to one was added a drachm of white wine vinegar, to the other an equal quantity of ſpring water. Thus with reſpect to dilution they were preciſely in the ſame circumſtances. A tea ſpoonful of the ſolution of *ſal martis* was then mixed with each of them. The portion which contained the vinegar, ſuffered no change of colour; the other inſtantly aſſumed a duſky hue. The ſame experiment was repeated with a very ſtrong triturated infuſion of the bark, and the reſult was nearly the ſame. As ſoon as a drachm of the vinegar was added to half an ounce of the infuſion, it changed the colour of it from a deep and reddiſh brown to a bright yellow; whilſt the ſame quantity of water, had no ſenſible diluting effect on the other portion with which

which it was mixed. The chalybeate ſolution, as in the former experiment, was then added. It produced no alteration in the portion with vinegar, but the other it changed into a perfect ink.

EXPERIMENT XXII.

To half an ounce of a ſtrong infuſion of galls were added two drachms of the ſolution of *ſal martis*. It preſently aſſumed the appearance of ink. Forty drops of the acid of vitriol reſtored it to its original colour. Thirty drops of the *ſp. c. c. vol.* renewed the inky blackneſs.

In theſe experiments it is obvious that an affinity ſubſiſts between acids, aſtringents, and bitters; and this ſuggeſted to me that they may poſſibly neutralize each other, and when combined together in due proportion, form what the chemiſts term a *tertium quid*. This important point, from which many uſeful inferences may be deduced, I attempted to afcertain in the following manner.

EXPERIMENT XXIII.

To half an ounce of a light infufion of the bark I added twenty drops of white wine vinegar. The acid and the bitter entirely corrected each other, and a new tafte was induced: after ftanding twelve hours, the mixture changed from a light yellow to a deep chocolate, and depofited a large brown fediment.

EXPERIMENT XXIV.

The fame quantity of vinegar was added to half an ounce of an infufion of Aleppo galls. The mixture was more auftere, and aftringent to the tafte than the infufion. After ftanding twelve hours, it depofited a floculent, whitifh fediment, and the liquor above became lefs auftere to the tafte than the fimple infufion itfelf.

EXPE-

EXPERIMENT XXV.

To equal quantities of ſpring water and of a ſtrong infuſion of gentian root, in ſeparate glaſſes, was added one drachm of white wine vinegar. The acid was entirely covered by the infuſion, but the ſpring water was manifeſtly ſour to the taſte. Sixty drops of the ſyrup of violets were then added to each. The infuſion ſuffered no change of colour; but the water aſſumed a light red, inclining ſomewhat to purple. Imagining that the deep colour of the infuſion prevented me from perceiving the action of the acid on the vegetable blue, I took the ſame quantity of old Mountain Wine, which was preciſely of the colour of the infuſion of gentian, and adding to it a drachm of vinegar, and ſixty drops of ſyrup of violets, I found a ſlight purple redneſs manifeſt itſelf about an hour after the mixture. The ſame experiment was repeated with a ſtrong infuſion of galls and diſtilled vinegar; but the reſult was not ſo obvious as in the former one, probably on account of the weaker powers of the acid employed.

EXPERIMENT XXVI.

Sir John Pringle hath proved that neutral ſalts reſiſt putrefaction with conſiderably leſs force, than the acids and alkalis of which they are compoſed. *Spiritus mindereri*, for inſtance, is not half ſo antiſeptic as the *ſal. c. c. vol:* and the common ſaline mixture of *ſal abſinth.* and *ſucc. limon.* is only three fourths as antiputreſcent as ſalt of wormwood ſeparately taken. *(a)* Dr. Macbride alſo hath demonſtrated, that acids and alkalis have the power of reſtoring ſweetneſs to putrid ſubſtances, but that when mixed together to the point of ſaturation, they loſe this property.

(a) Diſeaſes of the Army, Append. Exp. 5th. 9th.

property. (*a*) As there ſeems therefore, by the three foregoing experiments, to be an analogy between the combination of acids, aſtringents, or bitters, and acids and alkalis, curioſity induced me to purſue it; and I flattered myſelf, that though my attempts ſhould prove unſucceſsful, ſome uſeful facts might offer themſelves to my notice, and that my labour would not be without its reward.

An ounce and half of mutton, chopped very ſmall, was divided into five equal parts, and put into ſo many different phials. To the firſt, which was deſigned for a ſtandard, were added twelve drachms of ſpring water; to the ſecond, ten drachms of water, and two drachms of white wine vinegar; to the third, ten drachms of the decoction of the bark, and two drachms of vinegar; to the fourth, ten drachms of the decoction of

(*a*) Macbride's Eſſays, p. 129.

the bark; to the fifth, ten drachms of water and one ſcruple of bark finely powdered. The bottles were lightly ſtopped, and ſet in a ſand bath, the heat of which was regulated by a thermometer, and kept up to the hundreth degree of Farenheit's ſcale. In the night the lamp was ſuffered to go out. The changes as they occurred in the mixtures were carefully noted down, and were as follows.

The ſtandard phial in ſeven hours emitted many air bubbles, and was frothy at top; but had acquired no fetor; No. 4. the decoction of the bark was alſo a little frothy. The next day the ſtandard ſmelled offenſively, and No. 4. was juſt perceptibly tainted. The third day, the ſtandard was very fetid; No. 4. was evidently putrid. The fourth day, the ſtandard was ſo extremely offenſive that I removed it. No. 2. the vinegar and water, was not quite ſweet. No. 3. the decoc-

tion

tion of the bark and vinegar, was unchanged. No. 4. the decoction of the bark, was very fetid. No. 5. the powder of bark and water, was quite ſweet but a little mouldy. The 5th day, No. 2. the vinegar and water, was more offenſive than before. No. 4. the decoction of bark, was ſo putrid that I removed it. No. 3. and 5. were quite ſweet.

THE ſixth day. The phials were removed from the ſand bath yeſterday, on account of an accident which happened to the lamp; and they remained in the cold for twenty hours. This morning they were ſet by a warm fire. They were not much changed ſince the laſt examination.

THE ſeventh day. No. 2. the vinegar and water, was very offenſive, but had a peculiar fetor, totally different from the putrid ſmell of No. 1. and No. 4. It was therefore removed. No. 3. and No. 5. were ſweet.

The eighth day, No. 3. the decoction of bark and vinegar, was a little tainted. No. 5. the powder of bark and water, was perfectly ſweet, and did not become ſenſibly putrid till the thirteenth day from the time of mixture.

EXPERIMENT XXVII.

To an ounce of putrid ox gall were added an ounce and half of the decoction of bark, one drachm of the powder of bark, and three drachms of white wine vinegar. The putrid ſmell of the gall was entirely corrected; and the mixture continued ſweet fourteen days, though it was placed near a warm fire.

In the event of the two laſt experiments I was very much deceived. Before I undertook them I was almoſt fully perſuaded,

perſuaded, that there ſubſiſted a compleat analogy between the combination of acids, aſtringents or bitters, and acids and alkalis; and that the neutrals formed by the mixture of the former, like thoſe of the latter, would prove leſs antiſeptic than the ſubſtances ſeparately taken of which they are compoſed. This preconceived hypotheſis led me to ſuſpect the preſent practice of joining acids and the bark, in the cure of putrid diſeaſes, to be very improper, as I imagined they would counteract each others effect. To aſcertain this important point, I made the two preceding experiments with the moſt minute exactneſs; and though the reſult of them was the very reverſe of what I had ſuppoſed, I was neither mortified with my diſappointment at that time, nor am I now aſhamed to acknowledge it. In a long courſe of experiments, which are undertaken with ſome particular view, and not made at random, inſtances of ſelf deception frequently and unavoid-

unavoidably occur. And in general they happily ſerve as a ſpur to induſtry. We firſt conceive a fact, and then ſet about the demonſtration of it. If the trial ſucceed, our end is obtained, and for the moſt part we reſt ſatisfied. But if the proof fail, ſome unexpected phenomena oftentimes occur, which awaken our attention, and excite us to new purſuits. But whether this be the caſe or not, ſucceſs or diſappointment are equally uſeful in experimental enquiries; becauſe a negative truth may be of as much importance as a poſitive one.

The five laſt experiments furniſh, at leaſt, a preſumptive proof, that acids and aſtringents or bitters, neutraliſe each other. By mixture it appears their taſte and ſmell are altered; the acids loſe their property of ſtriking a red colour with ſyrup of violets; and their antiſeptic powers in combination, are double the ſum of them when ſeparately employed. The bark

bark likewife with vinegar [Exper. 27.] hath the power of reftoring fweetnefs to putrid fubftances, which it hath not alone, as Dr. Macbride affirms. *(a)* Sir John Pringle hath indeed afferted the contrary; but in his experiment the putrid alkali feems to have been wafhed off, not corrected, by repeated affufions of the decoction of the bark.

EXPERIMENT XXVIII.

FOUR pieces of calf fkin, frefh ftripped from the calf, and exactly of equal fizes, were immerfed, one in an ounce and half of the infufion of bark; the fecond in an ounce and half of the fame infufion, with two drachms of white wine vinegar; the third in an ounce and half of the infufion of Aleppo galls; the fourth in an ounce and half of the infufion of galls, with two drachms of vinegar.

At

(a) Macbride's Experimental Effays, p. 130

At the end of ſeven days they were taken out, and carefully examined. The pieces which had been immerſed in the infuſions of galls, and bark with vinegar, were much ſofter and more ſwoln, eſpecially in the middle, than the other two pieces: and the cuticle very eaſily ſeparated from the cutis, which was not the caſe with the others. So that the acid ſeemed greatly to diminiſh the aſtrictive powers of theſe two infuſions. The pieces were all ſo ſhriveled, that I could not eaſily meaſure them, nor determine which was the moſt contracted in ſize.

VINEGAR, it is well known, hath the property of ſoftening animal fibres in a very remarkable degree; and diluted with warm water, it is frequently employed as a reſolvent in external, topical inflammations. But when taken internally, or applied to any very ſenſible membrane, it acts as an aſtringent. Thus in the mouth

it

it corrugates the tongue and palate, and induces a paleneſs in the lips, by contracting the ſmall capillary arteries which run upon their ſurface. And when injected into the *vagina*, it proves an excellent remedy in the *fluor albus*, but requires in ſome caſes, to be diluted with water, otherwiſe it would be too ſuddenly aſtrictive and corroborant. On what principles it is that it produces ſuch oppoſite effects on the dead and living fibre, it would be difficult with certainty to determine. Perhaps its aſtringent property may depend upon its ſtimulus, which can only exert itſelf on the *ſolida viva*; as the ſimple ſolids are the proper ſubjects of its reſolvent power. But although the preceding experiments clearly prove, that vinegar in combination with aſtringents, diminiſhes their corrugating effects on the dead fibre; I would by no means infer, that its action is the ſame when applied to the living fibre, or that acids and the bark are improperly exhibited

exhibited together in the cure of hemorrhages. From the 24th experiment it appears, that the infuſion of galls is rendered much more auſtere to the taſte by the addition of vinegar; and it is not improbable, that its aſtrictive power as a medicine is increaſed in the ſame proportion. For I apprehend that the taſte, with reſpect to the operation of this claſs of vegetables on the body, is the leaſt fallacious teſt of aſtringency. I term it the leaſt fallacious teſt, becauſe it will be ſhewn afterwards, in the ſucceeding ſection, that neither the taſte, nor the property of ſtriking a black colour with chalybeates, nor yet the power of hardening animal fibres, whether ſeparately or collectively taken, are certain criteria of the aſtringent power of a medicine on the living body. *(a)*

I SHALL

(a) WHEN the 28th experiment was made, it did not occur to me to try the effects of the mineral acids, in conjunction with the vegetable aſtringents. But I have

I SHALL conclude this section with a few obvious, practical inferences, from the foregoing observations and experiments.

1. IT is the opinion of a very eminent physician, that the bark, when taken in substance, disagrees with weak stomachs, on account of its fermenting quality. *(a)* But I think the 16th. 17th. and 18th. experiments, which prove its remarkably slow solubility, furnish a better explanation of the fact. When the stomach is overloaded with a dose of the *cortex* in powder, a sense of weight and oppression, not of flatulency or distension, is for the most part complained of. And it is a common, and I believe useful

have since found by an experiment, made with the decoction of the bark and elixir of vitriol, that the astrictive power of the former is much increased by the addition of the latter.

(a) Pringle's Dis. Army. Append. p. 66.

uſeful practice, to join aromatics with the bark, and that doubtleſs with a view to ſtimulate the digeſtive powers, and quicken its paſſage through the *primæ viæ*. For as it is evident from the experiments of Sir John Pringle himſelf, that they are of a very fermentable nature, they cannot correct, but muſt rather promote that tendency in the *cortex*, and add to the uneaſineſs which it occaſions by the freſh generation of air. But the beſt proof that the bark is not ſo prone to run into fermentation, and that it is in ſome ſtomachs almoſt indigeſtible, is the caſe of a patient of the late Dr. Alſton, who vomited up a doſe of it almoſt unchanged eight days after taking it. *(a)* A very ingenious friend of mine hath remarked in the courſe of his practice, that the bark in ſubſtance is leſs oppreſſive when given in draughts, than either in the form of a bolus or electuary.

(a) Cullen's Lect. on the Mat. Medica.

electuary. A considerable quantity of unfixed air, he says, adheres to the particles of the powder, which occasions disturbances when carried into the stomach. By combining the *cortex* with any liquid, this air is in a great measure, he thinks, separated, as appears by the bubbles which are formed, and the frothyness which is produced during the act of mixture.

THE fact is curious, and I doubt not perfectly true; but the explanation of it is more plausible than satisfactory. The bark when administered in draughts, is generally mixed with some agreeable aromatic water, which renders it more palatable, dilutes it in the stomach, and by its grateful warmth promotes the more speedy digestion of it. But when given in a bolus or electuary, which are for the most part made up with syrups, it is peculiarly nauseous, owing probably to the unpleasant combination of sweet and bitter. And it is a common obſervation, that what is diſguſting to the palate, is generally offenſive to the ſtomach. The more ſolid form of theſe two preparations is likewiſe unfavourable to quick ſolution. Soap pills have been known to paſs through the whole inteſtinal canal undiſſolved. In a weak ſtate therefore of the ſtomach and bowels, we need not wonder that a large maſs of an electuary of the bark, ſhould lie long unchanged, and prove very oppreſſive.

2. As it appears from ſeveral experiments, that bitters have the property of neutraliſing acids, their uſe in acidities of the firſt paſſages is very obvious. In ſuch caſes indeed they may be conſidered as indicated on a double account, to correct the diſeaſe when preſent, and by their bracing and corroborant effects to remove the cauſe, and prevent the return of it. When given with ſuch intentions,

they

they ſhould be infuſed in brandy, or in ſome of the ſtronger wines. It has been long the practice to exhibit bitters in icterical complaints, as a ſubſtitute for the bile. But though with this view, they are improperly employed, as being antiſeptic, retarders, and moderators of fermentation, and conſequently very different from the bile, which is poſſeſſed of all the oppoſite qualities; yet I cannot join with a very celebrated phyſician in opinion, that they do little or no ſervice in the jaundice. (a) This diſeaſe, when it has been of ſome ſtanding, is almoſt always accompanied with loſs of appetite and indigeſtion, and with acidities and flatulencies in the *primæ viæ*. The ſtomach and bowels, from the defect of bile, are deprived of their uſual *ſtimulus*, their periſtaltic motion is impaired, and the food, by long ſtagnation, runs with violence through its ſucceſſive ſtages of fermentation.

(a) Pringle's Append. to Diſ. Army. p. 72.

mentation. In this ſtate of the diſtemper, the *ſaliva* and *ſuccus pancreaticus* probably acquire a morbid diſpoſition, and inſtead of aſſiſting digeſtion, and checking the generation of air, ſerve rather to injure the one, and promote the other, increaſing the general tendency to ſourneſs and crudity. Under theſe circumſtances, evacuants, antacids, and antifermentatives are certainly indicated. Vomits and purgatives anſwer the firſt, and bitters the two laſt intentions. The former are adapted to remove the cauſe of the diſeaſe; the latter only to palliate ſome of its moſt troubleſome ſymptoms. In this view however they are of importance; and the uſe of them ſhould by no means be diſcouraged.

3. IN a poſthumous work of the learned Dr. Boerhaave, publiſhed by his pupil Van Eems, it is aſſerted, that the deleterious effects of ſcammony, colocynth, and ſpurge, are corrected by vinegar. *(a)* Theſe

(a) Boerhaave de Morb. Nor. Cap. de Paralyſi.

Theſe are all vegetable bitters, and probably the action of the acid conſiſts in neutraliſing them. If this be the caſe, the uſe of vinegar as an antidote, may perhaps be more extenſive than is commonly ſuppoſed. For many of thoſe ſubſtances, which on account of their virulent and pernicous effects on the body, are termed poiſons, have a conſiderable degree of bitterneſs; as may be inſtanced in the *lauro ceraſus*, *nux vomica*, *helleborus*, *nicotiana*, *camphor*, *opium*, *euphorbium*, *aſarum*, *bryonia*, *coloquintida*, *elaterium*, *chelidonium majus*, &c. And it is at leaſt as probable, that their noxious qualities reſide in their bitter, as in any other part of their compoſition. (a)

I 3 4. Dr.

(a) On communicating this conjecture to my ingenious and learned friend Dr. Dobſon of Liverpool, he furniſhed me with the two following experiments in confirmation of it.

EXPE-

4. Dr. Hillary, in his treatiſe on the Yellow Fever of the Weſt India iſlands, diſcom-

EXPERIMENT I.

" May 21, 1764. Twelve grains of Opium, diſſolved in half an ounce of water, were given to a Pointer Bitch, which weighed twenty five pounds and two ounces. The natural ſtate of her pulſe was from 110 to 115 pulſations in a minute; and it ſhould be premiſed, that in making the following experiments, I never examined the pulſe, but after ſhe had been in my room 15 or 20 minutes, and was either aſleep or lay at reſt.

Soon after giving her the opium, ſhe looked heavy; ſlavered a great deal; and appeared to be much offended with the taſte of the opium.

When at liberty, ſhe went out into the open air, but was dull and moved ſlowly.

One hour after; Pulſe 75. Very uneaſy and diſtreſſed. An univerſal rigor and trembling every five or ſix ſeconds.

Two hours after; Pulſe 60. Had run out into the ſtreet for half an hour; head rather giddy, with an unſteadineſs in her gait; complains and groans frequently; heavy, but does not ſleep much; ſlavers a great deal.

Three hours after; Pulſe 59. In other reſpects much the ſame.

Five hours after; Pulſe 60. Had been in the open air for more than an hour; rather ſtaggered as ſhe went down ſome ſteps; frequently kept her head very erect, but

discommends the use of the bark in that disease, chiefly on account of its disa-

I 4 greement

but not steady; slept very little; lost all her playfulness; slavers; refuses to eat bread; offended with the taste of the opium; and has still the tremblings and twitchings.

EIGHT HOURS AFTER; Pulse 80. More brisk, and seems to be coming to herself again.

TWELVE HOURS AFTER; Pulse 86. Had followed the servant for more than a mile; still more herself.

SIXTEEN HOURS AFTER; Pulse 113. Not much different from her usual appearance.

EXPERIMENT II.

May 28th, 1764. Twelve grains of opium dissolved as in the former experiment, and with the addition of 30 drops of the acid elixir of vitriol, were given to the same Pointer. Much offended with the taste; foams and slavers.

ONE HOUR AFTER; Pulse 90. Slavers very little; alert as usual. As she lay asleep in my room, she had a little rigor and trembling.

TWO HOURS AFTER; Pulse 85. There were now given her 20 drops of the elixir of vitriol in an ounce of water; slavered a little after this.

THREE HOURS after; Pulse 80. The slavering soon ceased; is not near so much offended with the taste of the opium as in the former experiment. Rigor and trembling very observable, but only when asleep: 30 drops of elixir

greement with the ſtomachs of his patients. He acknowledges however, that it is ſtrongly indicated, and ſeems to lament, that even under the pleaſanteſt form it cannot be retained. But from the 27th experiment I ſhould conclude, that

elixir of vitriol were now given; and one hour after this, 20 drops more; ſo that ſhe has had in all 100 drops of the elixir of vitriol, within the four hours.

Five hours after; Pulſe 95. Briſk; ſome of the twitchings, but only when aſleep.

Eight hours after; Pulſe 120. Not much different from her uſual appearance; ſome very ſlight twitchings as ſhe lay aſleep.

Theſe and ſome other experiments were made, in order to aſcertain the efficacy of acids in counteracting the deleterious qualities of opium. When an over doſe of opium has remained in the ſtomach for ſome time, the ſenſibility of that organ is almoſt entirely deſtroyed, ſo that the moſt active emetics are ineffectual to evacute the poiſon. It is a matter of conſequence therefore in this caſe, to know what claſs of medicines we may next have recourſe to, with the greateſt probability of ſucceſs. As the opium cannot be rejected from the ſtomach, relief is only to be expected from ſuch remedies as will change the nature of the opium itſelf: and how far this end is to be attained by the liberal uſe of acids, the reader may judge by comparing theſe two experiments."

that it would ſit tolerably eaſy, or at leaſt that it would not be rejected, if it were combined with the vegetable acids. A redundance and corruption of the bile are the pathognomonic ſymptoms of this fever; and notwithſtanding the incredible evacuation of it in the firſt ſtage of the diſtemper, there ſtill continues through the whole courſe of it, both an inordinate ſecretion of that humour in the liver, and a depravation of it in the firſt paſſages. In ſuch circumſtances, the bark given by itſelf cannot fail to diſagree; for when mixed with putrid gall, it is obſerved greatly to increaſe the fetor of it. *(a)* But when joined with acids, which have the power of neutralizing the corrupted bile, as will hereafter be proved, it can occaſion no diſturbance, and muſt be highly ſerviceable, not only as an antiſeptic, but alſo as a corrobo-

(a) Macbride's Eſſays, p. 140.

corroborant. The truth of this remark is confirmed, even by the practice of Dr. Hillary himſelf, who exhibits an infuſion of ſnake root as a ſubſtitute for the *cortex*, and accompanies it with the elixir of vitriol.

SEC-

SECTION III.

HAVING frequently obſerved, during the courſe of my experiments, that the aſtringency and bitterneſs of vegetables are diſtinct and ſeparate properties, I was deſirous of tracing their differences, and of aſcertaining the proportion which they reciprocally bear to each other. To this end I made a variety of trials, and though not with all the ſucceſs that I wiſhed or expected, yet as they throw ſome light on this intricate ſubject, I ſhall here faithfully relate ſuch of them, as were moſt concluſive and ſatisfactory.

EXPERIMENT XXIX.

To equal quantities of ſtrong infuſions of

of Aleppo galls and gentian root, were added two drachms of a ſolution of green vitriol. The infuſion of galls inſtantly ſtruck a deep, inky blackneſs: that of the gentian root was unaltered in colour. The former it is well known is very ſlightly, the latter very intenſely bitter.

EXPERIMENT XXX.

To equal quantities of ſtrong infuſions of rue, wormwood, gentian, green tea, bohea tea, biſtort, and galls, was added a tea ſpoonful of the ſolution *ſal martis*. The galls aſſumed the deepeſt black; the infuſion of biſtort was next in degree; then followed the green and bohea tea, between which I could perceive no difference; the tinge of the wormwood and rue was a little deepened, but the gentian was unaltered. Their degrees of bitterneſs were in the following order; 1. gentian. 2. wormwood. 3. rue. 4. green and bohea tea. 5. biſtort. 6. galls.

6. galls. The two laſt were very ſlightly bitter. Twenty drops of white wine vinegar diſcharged the colour, induced by the green vitriol on the infuſions of rue and wormwood: a hundred drops conſiderably diminiſhed the blackneſs of the infuſions of galls, biſtort, and bohea tea. But the firſt, after ſtanding twenty four hours, recovered its inky colour, and a number of fine, jet black flakes floated about in it, without ſubſiding: The colouring particles of the two laſt, much diminiſhed in their blackneſs, ſunk to the bottom of the glaſſes. Twenty drops of oil of vitriol entirely diſcharged the black colour of the green tea, and it continued clear and pellucid.

EXPERIMENT XXXI.

To determine the comparative antiſeptic powers of bitters and aſtringents, I put into ten phials marked 1. 2. 3. &c. a drachm and half of mutton, which had been

been kept ſeveral days, but was perfect-ly ſweet. To the firſt, which was intended for a ſtandard, was added an ounce of ſpring water; to the ſecond, an ounce of a cold infuſion of green tea; to the third, an ounce of an infuſion of common wormwood; to the fourth, an ounce of the decoction of the bark; to the fifth, an ounce of the infuſion of galls; to the ſixth, an ounce of a cold infuſion of the bark; to the ſeventh, an ounce of a cold infuſion of rue; to the eighth, an ounce of a cold infuſion of biſtort; to the ninth, an ounce of a cold infuſion of bohea tea; to the tenth, an ounce of a cold infuſion of gentian. By miſtake only the five firſt phials were placed in the ſand bath, the other five were left in my ſtudy window, which has a northern aſpect. I was called from home, and was abſent three days and a half. On my return, I found No. 1. 2. 3. 4. the ſtandard, the green tea, the wormwood, and the decoction of bark, were

were all putrid, but in different degrees, according to the order in which they are marked down. No. 5. the infuſion of galls was unchanged. The mixtures, which had been left in my ſtudy window, were quite ſweet; but they ſeemed to have ſome little fermentative motion in them. They were placed in the ſand bath, and the next day I examined them. No. 7. the infuſion of rue was very offenſive. No. 6. the infuſion of bark was putrid, but in a leſs degree than the rue. No. 5. 8. 9. 10. were all ſweet. The day following No. 9. the infuſion of bohea tea was very putrid. No 8. the infuſion of biſtort was a little tainted. No. 5. the infuſion of galls, and No. 10. the infuſion of gentian, continued ſweet; and as they remained unchanged ſeveral days longer, I removed them from the ſand bath, fully ſatisfied with the proof of their ſtrong antiſeptic powers.

EXPER-

EXPERIMENT XXXII.

Eight pieces of calf ſkin, juſt ſtripped from the calf, and exactly of equal ſizes, viz. two inches long, and an inch broad, were ſeverally immerſed in an ounce and half of each of the following preparations. 1. *decoct. cort. peruv.* 2. cold infuſion of the bark. 3. cold infuſion of galls. 4. cold infuſion of gentian. 5. cold infuſion of green tea. 6. cold infuſion of bohea tea. 7. cold infuſion of rue. 8. Simple water as a ſtandard. At the expiration of a week, they were taken out and examined. The piece in the water was ſoft and putrid. That in the infuſion of rue was ſweet but ſoft. Thoſe in the infuſions of green and bohea tea, were hard and curled up; nor did there appear to be any ſenſible difference between them. The infuſion of gentian ſeemed to poſſeſs no inconſiderable degree of aſtringency;

gency; for the piece of ſkin immerſed in it, was nearly as hard, and as much ſhriveled, as thoſe in the infuſions of green and bohea tea. The decoction and infuſion of the bark were, to all appearance, alike in their degree of aſtringency, which was rather greater than that of tea, but much inferior to the galls.

THIS experiment affords a ſtriking proof, of the difference between the action of a medicine on the dead, and on the living fibre. Tea, when applied to the former, is manifeſtly aſtringent; and yet when received into the ſtomach, it is highly debilitating and relaxant, and the immoderate uſe of it is attended with the moſt pernicious effects. It is curious to obſerve the revolution which hath taken place, within this century, in the conſtitutions of the inhabitants of Europe. Inflammatory diſeaſes more rarely occur, and, in general, are much leſs rapid and violent in their progreſs, than formerly. *(a)* Nor do they admit of the ſame antiphlogiſtic method of cure, which was practiſed with ſucceſs a hundred years ago. The experienced Sydenham makes forty ounces of blood, the mean quantity to be drawn in the acute Rheumatiſm; whereas this diſeaſe, as it now appears in the London Hoſpitals, will not bear above half that evacuation Vernal intermittents are frequently cured by a vomit and the bark, without venæſection; which is a proof, that, at preſent, they are accompanied with fewer ſymptoms of inflammation, than they were wont to be. This advantageous change however is more than counterbalanced, by the introduction of a numerous claſs of nervous ailments, in a great meaſure unknown

(a) THE decreaſe in the violence of inflammatory diſeaſes may, perhaps in part, be aſcribed to the preſent improved method of treating them. Moderate evacuations, cool air, aceſcent diet, and the liberal uſe of ſaline and antimonial medicines, are better adapted to check the progreſs of fevers, than copious bleedings, ſtimulating purgatives, and profuſe ſweats, excited by *theriaca* or mithridate.

known to our anceſtors, but which now prevail univerſally, and are complicated with almoſt every other diſtemper. The bodies of men are enfeebled and enervated, and it is not uncommon to obſerve very high degrees of irritability, under the external appearance of great ſtrength and robuſtneſs. The hypochondria, palſies, cachexies, dropſies, and all thoſe diſeaſes which ariſe from laxity and debility, are in our days endemic every where; and the hyſterics, which uſed to be peculiar to the women, as the name itſelf indicates, now attacks both ſexes indiſcriminately. It is evident, that ſo great a revolution could not be effected, without the concurrence of many cauſes; but amongſt theſe, I apprehend, the preſent general uſe of tea holds the firſt and principal rank. The ſecond place may perhaps be allotted to exceſs in ſpirituous liquors. This pernicious cuſtom, in many inſtances at leaſt, owes its riſe to the former, which by the lowneſs and depreſſion of ſpirits it occaſions, renders it almoſt neceſſary to have recourſe to what is cordial and exhilerating. And hence proceed thoſe odious and diſgraceful habits of intemperance, with which too many of the ſofter ſex of every degree, are now, alas! chargeable.

FROM the 27th. and 29th. experiments it appears, that green and bohea tea are equally bitter, ſtrike preciſely the ſame black tinge with green vitriol, and are alike aſtringent on the ſimple fibre. From this exact ſimilarity in ſo many circumſtances, one ſhould be led to ſuppoſe, that there would be no ſenſible diverſity in their operation on the living body. But the fact is otherwiſe. Green tea is much more ſedative and relaxant than bohea; and the finer the ſpecies of tea, the more debilitating and pernicious are its effects, as I have frequently obſerved in others, and experienced

enced in myſelf. *(a)* This ſeems to be a proof, that the miſchiefs aſcribed to this oriental vegetable, do not ariſe from the warm vehicle by which it is conveyed into the ſtomach, but chiefly from its own peculiar qualities. *(b)* And theſe qualities probably accompany the highly flavoured parts of the leaves, and depend upon the nicety and care obſerved in the

 collection

(a) I HAVE now under my care a lady, of a moſt delicate conſtitution, who has been long ſubject to a *profluvium menſium*, to frequent diarrhœas, and to copious and ſudden diſcharges of urine. Bohea tea, of a moderate degree of ſtrength, ſeldom fails to check the *catamenia*, and ſhe has uſed it for this purpoſe ten or twelve months. Green tea, whenever ſhe drinks it, produces tremors, anxiety, and a large flux of urine, which ſhe voids in the quantity of two or three pints at once. The bladder is not over diſtended, previous to the diſcharge; but ſhe feels (to uſe her own expreſſion) as if the urine flowed from all parts of her body to the kidneys, during the time of micturition. It ſhould be remarked that this lady never uſes bohea tea, but at a particular period, medicinally.

(b) THEÆ infuſum, nervo muſculove ranæ admotum, vires motrices minuit, perdit.

Smith Tentamen Inaug. de actione muſculari, p. 46. exp. 36.

collection and preparation of them. When fresh gathered, they are said to be narcotic, and to disorder the senses; and the Chinese cautiously abstain from the use of them, till they have been kept for twelve months. (a) It is remarkable that only one species of the tea plant is yet discovered, and that all the varieties of this dietetic article of commerce, are owing either to the difference of climate, or to the diversity in the method of curing it. The fine green teas, which are the first crop of the shrub, are gathered with the utmost caution, and dried with the gentlest heat, that their perishable flavour may be preserved. The bohea teas are more hastily exsiccated, and even slightly parched over the fire, by

(a) Neumann's Chemistry, p. 376.

A GENTLEMAN of veracity, who commanded an East India ship several voyages to China, says that the Chinese rarely drink the green tea; and that those who drink it to excess, are thrown thereby into a diabetes, or become tabid, and die emaciated.

Vid. Med. Museum, vol. 2. p. 51.

by which they acquire that brown colour which diſtinguiſhes them. And as their more volatile parts are diſſipated by this management, they become proportionably leſs injurious to the nervous ſyſtem.

An ingenious phyſician, who has done me the honour to adopt my ſentiments, and to quote my arguments againſt the uſe of tea, in his Inaugural Diſſertation, publiſhed at Leyden, 1769, has confirmed my teſtimony by the following experiments. (a) " He injected into the cavity of

(a) Dissertatio Medica Inauguralis, ſiſtens Obſervationes ad vires Theæ pertinentes, auctore J. C. Lettſom. As this Diſſertation is proabbly but in few hands, the following extracts from it, which contain his experiments at large, may not be unacceptable to my learned reader.

EXPERIMENTUM I.

Sumpsi infuſionis Theæ viridis, & Boheæ, liquoris poſt diſtillationem ſuperſtitis; nec non aquæ ſimplicis cujuſlibet æqualem quantitatem, & in quemlibet liquorem, in vaſe ſuo contentum, immiſi drachmas duas carnis bovis, ante duos dies mactati.

Caro bovina, immerſa in aquam ſimplicem, poſt quadraginta octo horas corrupta, putridaque devenerat; dum portiones

of the abdomen, and into the cellular membrane of a frog, about three drachms of

portiones carnis in reliquas tres Theæ infusiones immissæ, post septuaginta demum horas putredinis indicia monstrabant.

EXPERIMENTUM II.

Viridis atque Boheæ Theæ, saturatis infusionibus addidi æquales portiones salis martis, & protinus utrumque infusum colorem æqualem, profunde nigrum, adquirebat.

Ex enarratis experimentis tuto concludere licet, Theam & viridem & Boheam manifesta virtute antiseptica, ac adstringente in fibris mortuis, & vi vitali carentibus, gaudere; verumtamen propria, & etiam aliorum, experientia edoctus, certus scio, eam, in ventriculum ingestam, præsertim in subjectis tenerioris & delicatioris compagis solidæ, insignem potestatem relaxantem exserere.

1. Potum hunc usitatum forma aquæ calidæ, aut fervidæ, sumendi mos invaluit, & inde nonnulli deducere voluerunt effectum, atque vim debilitantem potius huic vehiculo, quam herbæ ipsi tribuendam esse. Verum enimvero omnia experimenta, curiosius capta, in eo consentiunt, quod Thea viridis, & præcipue illa, quæ subtilissimum, atque maxime penetrabilem, spargit odorem, multo majori gradu virtutem relaxantem, quam Thea Bohea dicta, præstet. Id quod animum mihi addidit investigationes inceptas ulterius atque plenius prosequendi.

2. Hoc fine libram dimidiam herbæ Theæ viridis optimæ notæ, & admodum fragrantis, cum aqua simplici distillavi,

of a highly ſcented, and pellucid liquor, which exhibited no ſigns of aſtringency, nor

diſtillavi, atque aquæ inſigniter odoratæ, pellucidæ, unciam unam, quæ nullum oleum in ſuperficiem excutiebat, neque ulla virtutis adſtrictivæ exhibuit indicia, elicui.

3. Eam partem liquoris, quæ finito ſtillicidio in vaſe diſtillatorio remanſit, ad extracti conſiſtentiam evaporavi, quod levem odorem, attamen ſaporem valde amarum adſtringentemque habebat. Extracti adquiſiti copia uncias quinque totidemque drachmas æquabat.

EXPERIMENTUM III.

In abdominis cavitatem, atque membranam celluloſam, ranæ injeci circiter tres drachmas aquæ ſtillatitiæ odoratæ. (No. 2.) Poſt viginti minuta alterum ranæ crus, ſeu pes poſterior, multum adficiebatur, dum parum mobilitatis, aut ſenſibilitatis, monſtrabat, quæ adfectio per quatuor horas perſeverabat, & rana in ſtatu torpido inſenſili univerſali ultra novem horas manebat, donec gradatim ad priſtinum vigorem rediret.

Simili ratione liquorem a deſtillatione Theæ viridis (No. 2.) ſuperſtitem, atque ulteriori evaporatione magis concentratum injeci, ſed inde nullum effectum ſenſibilem inductum vidi.

EXPERIMENTUM IV.

Nervis Iſchiaticis ranæ denudatis, atque cavitati abdominis, aquam ſtillatitiam fragrantem (No. 2. & Exp. III.) adplicui, intra dimidiam horam extremitates poſteriores,

nor had any oil floating on its ſurface, diſtilled from half a pound of fine hyſon tea. In twenty minutes the hinder extremities of the frog were ſtrongly affected, and continued ſo four hours, whilſt the animal remained in a torpid, inſenſible ſtate upwards of nine hours, and then recovered by degrees its former vigour. He made the ſame experiment with the *reſiduum*,

riores penitus paralyticæ inſenſileſque deveniebant, & poſt horæ circiter ſpatium rana vivere deſiit.

Liquorem a diſtillatione reſiduum (No. 2. & Exper. III.) eadem ratione alii ranæ admovi, ſed nullos inde natos obſervare potui effectus ſedantes, immo virtutem magis ſtimulantem, quam ſedativam, præſtare videbatur.

Extractum (No. 3.) in aqua ſolutum, & ſub iiſdem conditionibus, iiſdem partibus admotum, nullum effectum ſenſibilem produxit.

4. Experimenta hæc enumerata nullis commentariis egent. Extra omnem dubitationis aleam ponere videntur, quod effectus Theæ ſedativus & relaxans a principio odorato, volatili, aromatico, potius, quam ab aqua calida dependeat. (No. 1.) Non pauca utriuſque ſexus ſubjecta mihi innotuerunt, quæ maxima moleſtia & anxietate torquebantur, quotieſcumque unum tantum poculum infuſi Theæ potaverant, quæ tamen, conſortio gratificandi ergo, aquam calidam loco, & more, infuſionis Theæ, ſine ullo effectu incommodante hauſerunt.

residuum, left after diſtillation, which produced no ſenſible effect.

He applied to the iſchiadic nerves of a frog, when laid bare by diſſection, and to the cavity of the *abdomen*, the ſame ſcented, diſtilled liquor mentioned above. In half an hour the hinder extremities became totally paralytic, and about an hour afterwards the frog died. The *reſiduum*, after diſtillation, was applied to another frog under the ſame circumſtances, but ſeemed to produce rather an aſtrictive, and ſtimulating, than narcotic effect. He prepared an extract from this *reſiduum*, which being diſſolved in water, and uſed in a ſimilar manner, had no viſible operation.

These experiments demonſtrate, that the pernicious effects of tea depend on its more volatile parts, which are diſſipated in a great degree by long keeping, by haſty drying, or by reducing it to the orm of an extract. I have ſeen and taſted of of ſuch an extract, made in the Eaſt Indies, which though bitter and aſtringent, was by no means unpalatable. A preparation of this kind, diſſolved in hot water, would be a good ſubſtitute for the leaves of the tea plant.

But however cogent the objections may be, againſt the general and too frequent uſe of tea, candour obliges me to acknowledge, that it is capable of being applied to very important, medicinal purpoſes. From its ſedative power, and the weakneſs which it ſuddenly induces, it might be adminiſtered with advantage in ardent and inflammatory fevers, in order to abate the force, and leſſen the inordinate action of the *vis vitæ*. In ſuch caſes it ſhould be given either in ſubſtance, or in ſtrong infuſion; and beſides allaying the troubleſome ſenſations of heat and thirſt, which are the conſtant concomitants of thoſe diſtempers, it would probably ſerve as a good ſubſtitute for ſome of the uſual evacuations. And thus

inſtead

inſtead of producing watchfulneſs, which is a common effect aſcribed to it in weak habits, it would in all likelihood prove the ſafeſt and moſt ſalutary opiate. After a full meal, when the ſtomach is oppreſſed, the head pained, and the pulſe beats high, tea is a grateful diluent, and agreeable ſedative. And as ſtudious, ſedentary men are particularly ſubject to indigeſtion and the head ach, it is on this account juſtly ſtiled "the poet's friend." Other uſes to which tea is applicable might eaſily be pointed out; but I have already made too long a digreſſion.

THE 29th. experiment affords a further proof, that the aſtringent parts of the *cortex* are as well extracted by maceration as by decoction. But I am inclined to think from this, and many other trials, that the aſtrictive quality of this medicine is not ſo great as it is commonly reputed to be: and conſequently the prejudice entertained againſt the uſe of it, in caſes where powerful aſtrin-

aſtringents are ſuppoſed to be contraindicated, is without ſufficient foundation. Thus it hath been a commonly received rule not to exhibit the bark in intermittents, before the diſeaſe be in ſome meaſure ſpontaneouſly abated; and then to adminiſter it only in the intervals of the fits. *(a)* But this extreme caution, as it took its riſe at firſt from falſe theory, is found by later experience to be in moſt inſtances unneceſſary; and the *cortex* is now frequently given with the utmoſt ſafety and ſucceſs, after previous evacuations, not only at the commencement of the diſorder, but even juſt before the acceſſion of the cold fit. This was the common method of exhibiting the bark when it was firſt introduced into Europe. *(b)* But Sydenham informs us, that

(a) Curandum eſt ante omnia ne præmature nimis hic cortex ingeratur, ante ſcilicet quam morbus ſuo ſe marte aliquantiſper protriverit.

Sydenham. Opera. p. 57.

(b) Tho. Bartholin. Hiſt. Anatom. Medic. Cent. 5. p. 108.

that not long after it came into disuse, for two reasons; "*Primò quia paucis horis ante adventum paroxysmi, pro recepto id temporis more, exhibitus, ægro nonnunquam è medio tolleret. Funestior hic pulveris exitus, quamvis oppidò rarus, medicos tamen paulo cordatiores ab ejus usu meritò retraxit. Secundò quia æger ope pulveris, à paroxysmo aliàs invasuro liberatus, quod plerumque eveniebat, tamen intra dies* 14. *recidivam ut plurimum pateretur, in morbo scilicet recenti, necdum temporis cursu suoque marte commitigato.* (*a*) The last objection would have been obviated by a longer use of the bark; the first is totally without foundation. For the very few instances of mortality (Sydenham only enumerates two) which immediately succeeded the exhibition of the *cortex*, were not to be ascribed to the operation of the powder, but to the violence of the cold fit, which without doubt would have carried off the patients, had no medicine been

(*a*) Sydenhami Opera, p. 265.

been adminiſtered. For the natural tendency of the bark is to moderate, and not to increaſe the force of the paroxyſms. And ſo far is it from producing obſtructions, when given, with proper precautions, at the beginning of intermittents, that it effectually prevents them, by putting a ſpeedy ſtop to the diſeaſe, the continuance of which in weak habits is the true cauſe of their formation. " I am convinced, ſays Mr. Cleghorn in his excellent treatiſe on the diſeaſes of Minorca, that the unhappy *metaſtaſes*, which ſome have obſerved to follow the uſe of the bark, are exceedingly rare, and ought rather to be aſcribed to other cauſes than to this medicine. And I will venture to affirm, that more bad conſequences enſue from giving it too late than too ſoon; proſtration of ſtrength, ſudden death, or the moſt obſtinate chronic diſeaſes, being the uſual effects of delay. Whereas the worſt that commonly happens from the too early uſe of it, is, that it does not at once reſtrain

ſtrain the paroxyſms like a charm, without any ſenſible evacuation, as it frequently does, when given after the fever has arrived naturally to its height, and begins to decline of its own accord." *(a)* In another part of his work, the ſame ingenious and accurate writer obſerves, "that the great advantage which accrues from the early uſe of the bark in tertians is, that it invigorates the powers of the body, prevents or removes the dangerous ſymptoms, and brings on a criſis ſoon, and with little diſturbance. Inſtead of ſuppreſſing any beneficial diſcharge, as ſome have aſſerted, we daily obſerve a laudable ſeparation in the urine, warm, profuſe, univerſal ſweats, plentiful bilious ſtools, and ſometimes the hæmorrhoids, and menſes coming on after it has been uſed; though it effectually reſtrains the colliquative night ſweats, to which perſons weakened by tedious intermittents are incident." *(b)* Morton, who

L had

(a) Diſ. of Minorca, p. 206.

(b) Id. p. 189. 190.

had great experience of the innocence and efficacy of the *cinchona*, frequently preſcribed it without premiſing any evacuations; and he aſſerts, that after twenty five years practice, he never knew the leaſt bad conſequence enſue from its exhibition, nor had ever occaſion to repent the uſe of it. Dr. Lind informs us, that for three years paſt, he has annually preſcribed upwards of one hundred and forty pounds weight of bark, and never obſerved any bad ſymptoms which could with propriety be aſcribed to its uſe, except in two inſtances; in one of which it was ſuppoſed, though perhaps without ſufficient foundation, to have occaſioned an obſtruction of the *menſes*; in the other it produced a fit of ſuffocation in an aſthmatic patient, probably owing to its being given in ſubſtance, and in too large a doſe. *(a)* A celebrated profeſſor at Vienna has related a number of curious caſes, which fully evince the ſafety and efficacy

(a) Vid. Lind on the hot Climates. p. 294.

efficacy of the bark in ſemitertians, miliary, and malignant fevers. *Cortex peruvianus, vel declarante ſe malignitate, aliquamdiu poſt eruptionem exanthematum, vel cum ipſa exanthematum eruptione, vel etiam ante eruptionem eorum, vel ab ipſo morbi principio, ilico ſummo cum effectu datus eſt.* (a) In the inoculated ſmall-pox, inſtances of ſevere ague fits have been known to attack perſons, between the inſertion of the variolous matter, and the eruption of the pock, when the bark hath been given liberally and with ſucceſs, the principal buſineſs in the mean time ſuffering no injury or interruption. (b) And in the confluent ſmall-pox a very free uſe of it has not ſeemed, in a variety of caſes to have abated the ſpitting. (c) The retroceſſion of the morbid acrimony in the meaſles, is prevented

(a) *Vid.* De Haen Rat. Medend. vol. 1. p. 166. 264. 265. Paris Edit.

(b) *Vid.* Dimſdale on Inoculation. p. 12. *vid.* alſo the Monthly Review for Sep. 1766. p. 189.

(c) Medical Tranſact. vol. 1. p. 469.

vented by nothing more powerfully than by the *cortex*, which obviates the ſecondary fever, allays the cough, and continues the efflorefcence on the ſkin even to the twelfth day: whilſt the diſeaſe runs through its accuſtomed ſtages with the utmoſt regularity, and creates much leſs diſturbance and alarm than uſual. *(a)* I had lately under my care a patient, who was ſeized with an intermittent, whilſt he laboured under a ſevere *gonorrhœa*. The bark was given him in large quantity; and ſo far was it from ſuppreſſing the diſcharge, that it evidently increaſed it, and at the ſame time diminiſhed its virulence. The late Dr. Whytt informs us, that he ſwallowed in ſixteen days, near four ounces of it in ſubſtance, when he laboured under a catarrhous cough, without feeling any bad effects from its aſtringent quality. In a tertian, attended with a cough and ſpitting, after the uſe of vomits and ſome pectorals, he preſcribed

(a) Vid. Dr. Cameron's Paper, Med. Muſeum. p. 281.

ſcribed the *cortex* in the uſual quantity, without the breaſt being any way hurt by it. And he had repeated experience of its virtues in curing a hoarſeneſs after the meaſles, when unattended with a fever or difficult reſpiration. In the hooping cough alſo, when given early, he found it one of the beſt remedies. *(a)* The bark has been ſucceſsfully adminiſtered, in the quantity of a drachm, every three hours, to a woman two days after her delivery, without leſſening the *lochia*; and it has been frequently given to others during their *catamenia*, without the leaſt interruption of them. *(b)* Theſe facts ſufficiently evince the common apprehenſions concerning the aſtringent quality of the *cinchona* to be groundleſs. And it may be hoped, that all ſuch prejudices againſt the uſe of it will now vaniſh; as by its efficacy in the cure of ſcrophulous, glan-

(a) Whytt on Nervous Diſorders, p. 241.
(b) Medical Tranſact. vol. 1. p. 469.

dular tumours, it is proved to be even a powerful deobſtruent.

The property of ſtriking a black colour with green vitriol hath been aſcribed to all vegetable aſtringents without exception, and hath hitherto been regarded as an infallible teſt of their aſtringency. (a) But from the 29th. 30th. and 31ſt. experiments it is evident, that neither the one, nor the other are ſtrictly and univerſally true. For gentian appears to be endued with no inconſiderable aſtrictive power, and yet the infuſion of it ſuffers not the leaſt change from the addition of *ſal martis*. On the contrary, the infuſion of rue has no degree of aſtringency on the dead fibre, and yet it ſtrikes a faint black with green vitriol.

The

(a) The power by which they produce this blackneſs, ſays a celebrated chemiſt, and their aſtringency, or that by which they contract an animal fibre, and by which they contribute to the tanning of leather, ſeem to depend upon one and the ſame principle, and to be proportional to one another.

Lewis Com. Ph. Tech. p. 345.

The action of acids in neutralising vegetable bitters, as described in the last section, naturally led me to try their effects on the animal bitters. For this purpose I procured a quantity of fresh ox gall; but being prevented for several weeks, by various avocations, from pursuing my experiments, I found the gall at the end of that term extremely putrid. This accident pointed out to me a train of enquiries, somewhat different indeed from what I had at first proposed to myself, but which afterwards appeared to be much more interesting and important. I shall therefore make no apology for laying before the reader the result of them.

EXPERIMENT XXXIII.

Putrid ox gall, diluted with water, struck a green colour with syrup of violets, and sensibly effervesced with oil of vitriol, became turbid and of a light yellow colour. This experiment was repeated several times, and always with the ſame ſucceſs; ſo that I am pretty confident there muſt have been ſome error in that trial of Dr. Macbride's, from which he concludes, "that putrid ox gall ſhews no ſign of alkali; it neither efferveſceth with acids, nor does it change the colour of the blue juices; neither does it throw down any precipitate from the ſolution of corroſive ſublimate." *(a)* At firſt it occurred to me, that the miſtake into which this very ingenious and accurate experimentaliſt hath fallen, might ariſe from his not diluting the gall before he added the acid; by which the latter would be ſo inviſcated, as not to give ſufficiently evident ſigns of efferveſcence. But afterwards the curious obſervations of M. Gaber of Turin, concerning putrefaction, ſuggeſted to me a ſtill more probable ſource of fallacy to which Dr. Macbride was expoſed. That learned Italian hath clearly proved, "that the marks of alcaleſcence in putrifying animal

(a) Macbride's Eſſays, p. 101.

mal ſubſtances, are greater or leſs, or none at all, according to the time the experiment is made after the putrefaction begins; that ſuch ſubſtances, upon their firſt putrefaction, do not efferveſce with acids; that afterwards they efferveſce manifeſtly with them; but that at length they ceaſe from doing it, though the putrefaction ſtill continues." *(a)* Now it is not unlikely that Dr. Macbride's trial on the ox gall, was made, either before the volatile alcaline ſalt was formed, or after it was evaporated; as Sir John Pringle candidly acknowledges, happened in his experiments on putrid ſubſtances.

EXPERIMENT XXXIV.

To two drachms of putrid ox gall, diluted with half an ounce of water, were added twenty drops of *ol. vitriol.* A light yellow

(a) Vid. Miſcellanea Phil. Mathem. Societat. Privat. Taurinenſis: *vid.* alſo, Pringle on the Diſeaſes of the Army, Append. p. 125.

yellow cloud inſtantly formed itſelf, and the mixture ſlightly effervefced and became turbid: But though the peculiar fetor of the gall was deſtroyed, yet it emitted a ſtrong and diſagreeable ſmell, nor was its bitter taſte entirely corrected. Thirty drops rendered the mixture rather ſharp to the taſte; but ſtill the bitterneſs was perceptible: Nor did forty drops entirely deſtroy it, although that quantity made the mixture very ſour. After ſtanding a while, it aſſumed a deep green colour, a ſediment gradually formed itſelf, which in twenty four hours ſubſided to the bottom of the glaſs, and left the liquor above almoſt clear.

EXPERIMENT XXXV.

To the ſame quantity of putrid gall and water as in the former experiment, were added forty drops of white wine vinegar. The putrid fetor was entirely deſtroyed, and no other diſagreeable ſmell was produced in its room. The mixture became

became turbid, but in a leſs degree than the former with the oil of vitriol; and the effervеſcence was likewiſe much more obſcure. Sixty drops of vinegar ſeemed nearly to neutraliſe the gall. For though ſome ſmall degree of bitterneſs remained, it was very trifling, and by no means unpalatable.

EXPERIMENT XXXVI.

To a third glaſs of gall and water, mixed together in the above-mentioned proportions, were added forty drops of juice of lemons. The mixture became turbid, but the putrid ſmell was not perceptibly covered. A hundred and twenty drops neutraliſed the mixture, entirely correcting both the odour and taſte.

1. From theſe experiments may be deduced, the great utility of acids in all diſeaſes which either proceed from, or are accompanied by a redundance and depravation of the bile. And this ſeems

to be the caſe with moſt autumnal fevers, and in general with the epidemics of all hot countries, eſpecially where heat and moiſture are conjoined. For the former promotes the generation, and the latter the putrefaction of the bile. I have been aſſured, ſays Dr. Bryan Robinſon, by a very knowing butcher, that animals have leaſt bile in January, and moſt in July. *(a)* And Hippocrates hath obſerved, *Æſtate ſanguis adhuc viget, ſed et bilis exaltatur; per æſtatem etiam ac antumnum bile corpus abundat; autumno autem atra-bilis plurima eſt et fortiſſima.* *(b)* Mr. Cleghorn, in his account of the diſeaſes of Minorca, informs us, that he examined the bodies of near a hundred perſons who died of tertian fevers, and that he conſtantly found the *veſica fellea*, and the ſtomach and inteſtines overflowing with bilious matter. *(c)* The teſtimony of Proſper Alpinus

(a) Robinſon on the Operation of Medicines, p. 48.

(b) Hippocrates lib. de Nat. Hom. ſect. 14.

(c) Diſ. of Minorca, p. 165.

Alpinus likewiſe, ſtrongly confirms the truth of this obſervation. He ſays, *Alexandriæ autumno graſſantur febres peſtilentes multæ lethales, quæ fere quamplurimos invadunt. His vero notis pleræque dignoſcuntur: in principio enim vomitus multi, bilioſi ac virulenti obſervantur, á quibus cibum aſſumptum continere nequeunt, aſſiduiſque corporis agitationibus, inquietudinibuſque vexantur, ſtomachique angore anguntur. In pleriſque etiam obſervantur multæ, ſymptomaticæ dejectiones, liquidæ, bilioſæ, variæ, admodum ægré olentes ſive fætentes.* *(a)* The yellow fever of the Weſt Indies is always at the beginning attended with great ſickneſs, violent retching, and a copious diſcharge of bile. The vomiting recurs at ſhort intervals, often becomes almoſt inceſſant, and an incredible quantity of bile is ſometimes thrown up in a few hours. *(b)*

2. THE

(a) Alpinus de Medicin. Ægypt. lib. 1. cap. 14. p. 51.

(b) *Vid.* Hillary's Obſerv. on the Diſ. of Barbadoes *vid.* alſo Biſſet's Medical Eſſays and Obſervations.

2. The difference between the action of mineral and vegetable acids on putrid gall, as evidenced in the preceding trials, is deserving of particular notice. From the ignorance of this distinction, or want of attention to it, I believe the elixir of vitriol is often exhibited, when vinegar, or the sour juices of vegetables, would be much more serviceable. For though it is the common property of all acids to *correct* the putrid acrimony; yet the power of *sweetening* it, seems to be peculiar to those of the vegetable class. And as they are mildly aperient at the same time, they will not only neutralise the septic *colluvies*, which in some diseases lodges in the stomach and flexure of the *duodenum*, but will also gently tend to evacuate it: an advantage not to be expected from the mineral acids.

3. Mr. Browne Langrish, in his Modern Theory and Practice of Physic, relates the case of a poor man, who after eating

eating heartily of ſtale mutton, which he bought on account of its cheapneſs, was affected with vomiting and purging to a ſtrange degree, and in all reſpects ſeemed as if he had been poiſoned. Vinegar, diluted with water, contributed more than any other medicine towards his cure.

4. A TABLE ſpoonful of the juice of lemons, unmixed with any thing, is ſaid by an ingenious writer, (a) to have repeatedly proved a certain cure for a palpitation of the heart, after many of the medicines, called antihyſteric, had been tried in vain. This effect he aſcribes to an uncommon diſpoſition in the nerves of the ſtomach. But I think it is not improbable that the complaint proceeded from bilious acrimony, which the vegetable acid corrected and neutraliſed. This conjecture is confirmed by a ſimilar caſe which Dr. Biſſet hath related, of a middle aged gentleman who had a palpitation

(a) Whytt on Nerv. Diſorders, p. 372.

on of the heart, accompanied with ſome ſymptoms of the jaundice, and who was completely cured by drinking every evening weak rum punch, acidulated with the juice of Seville Oranges. (a)

5. I HAVE been lately informed by an ingenious practitioner, that he has ſeen four caſes of a ſuppreſſion of urine, ſuppoſed to ariſe from gravel in the kidneys, almoſt inſtantly removed by the juice of lemons. Not long after taking it the patient voided a quantity of ſabulous matter. In one caſe, a very painful chordee accompanied the complaint, which immediately yielded to the ſame medicine. All the patients were of bilious habits, and it is probable, the lemon juice reſolved the ſpaſms of the urinary paſſages, by correcting ſome putrid acrimony in the ſtomach, or by producing a grateful ſenſation in that organ. Sydenham recommends the juice of lemons, joined with manna,

(a) Biſſet's Medical Eſſays and Obſerv. p. 254.

manna, as a remedy for the gravel, and found in his own caſe that it rendered the purgative quicker in its action, and more agreeable to his ſtomach.

6. From the effect of acids on the gall, we may infer the reaſon why the immoderate uſe of them ſo much impairs digeſtion. The bile in its natural ſtate is a ſaponaceous fluid, abſolutely neceſſary to chylification; and whatever weakens its powers, muſt proportionably injure the due concoction and aſſimilation of our food. Hence the body is deprived of its proper nouriſhment and ſupport, the blood becomes vapid and watery, and a fatal cachexy unavoidably enſues. This has been the melancholy lot of many unfortunate perſons, who in order to reduce their exceſſive corpulency, have indulged themſelves in the too liberal uſe of vinegar.

7. It is not improbable that the acidi-

ties, to which infants are peculiarly ſubject, ariſe as much from the weakneſs of their biliary ſecretions, as from the aceſcency of their food. The liver of a child is extremely lax in its texture, and with reſpect to his bulk, is much larger than the liver of an adult: Hence the ſecretions of the one, will be proportionably greater than the ſecretions of the other. But though the bile flows copiouſly, yet the powers of nature in the ſtate of infancy are too feeble for its due preparation; and it is a mere watery, inert fluid, unfit for neutraliſing thoſe acidities, which in the more advanced ſtages of life, it is one part of its office to correct. And this, I apprehend, is a principal cauſe of their redundancy in the *primæ viæ* of children.

THE frequent opportunities which the preceding courſe of experiments afforded me, of obſerving the effects ariſing from the combination of green vitriol and aſtringents,

tringents, naturally led me to examine into the principles of INK. And as the ſubject is not only curious in itſelf, but alſo intereſting and important, from its relation to the arts of dying and ſtaining black, I was induced to inſtitute a new ſet of trials, in order to the more clear and accurate inveſtigation of it. That a ſolution of vitriol ſtrikes a deep black with vegetable aſtringents, is a fact univerſally known; but Dr. Lewis is almoſt the only chemiſt who hath attempted to explain it. He is of opinion that the colouring matter of ink is iron, extricated from its acid in a highly attenuated or divided ſtate, and combined with a peculiar ſpecies of matter contained in aſtringent vegetables. Acids, he ſays, deſtroy its blackneſs by rediſſolving the ferrugineous particles; and alkalis by uniting with the aſtringent matter, and precipitating the iron nearly in the ſame ochery ſtate, as they do from the ſimple acid ſolutions of the metal. (a)

But from the following experiments I think it will fully appear, that this very ingenious and uſeful chemiſt is miſtaken; and that the colouring matter of ink is iron, not extricated from, but in combination with an acid.

EXPERIMENT XXXVII.

To half an ounce of the decoction of galls, was added one grain of *ſal martis:* An inky blackneſs ſucceeded. Sixty drops of *ſp. c. c. vol.* diſcharged the black, and rendered the liquor thick and brown coloured. A hundred and twenty drops of oil of vitriol reſtored the blackneſs; two hundred again diſcharged it, and gave the ink a yellow caſt, inclining to green. This

(a) Lewis Comm. Ph. Tech. p. 348.

This experiment is illuſtrated by the following one.

EXPERIMENT XXXVIII.

ONE grain of green vitriol was diſſolved in half an ounce of ſpring water: forty drops of *ſp. c. c. vol.* were added; a greeniſh yellow ſediment formed itſelf, and preſently ſubſided to the bottom of the glaſs, with little white flakes, which I at firſt judged to be calcareous earth, ſeparated from the ſpring water by means of the volatile alkali. But the *ſp. c. c. vol.* mixed with the ſame water, produced no precipitation. Oil of vitriol was then dropped in, to the point of ſaturation. When the efferveſcence ceaſed, the whole ſediment was rediſſolved, and the mixture became quite clear.

EXPERIMENT XXXIX.

A PIECE of poliſhed iron was immerſed

in a cold infuſion of the bark, made with diſtilled water. In three hours the liquor was juſt perceptibly tinged with black. The piece of iron was then taken out, wiped clean, and again immerſed in another infuſion of the *cortex*, of equal ſtrength with the former, made with common ſpring water. In leſs than two hours, the infuſion aſſumed a deep purple colour, and the fluid in contact with the iron was of an inky blackneſs.

THIS experiment clearly proves, that an acid is neceſſary to the formation of ink. Spring water is generally impregnated with ſome of the mineral acids, in combination either with certain metallic ſubſtances, the foſſil alkali, or calcareous earth. The water employed in this trial, contained a conſiderable portion of ſelenitic ſalt; and hence it was capable of diſſolving the iron which was immerſed in it, and of forming with it a perfect *ſal martis*. This ſufficiently accounts for the

the deep purple hue which the infusion assumed. The distilled water was either not sufficiently pure, for I did not particularly examine it, or the *cortex*, which like all other vegetable substances, is of an acescent nature, communicated to it a slight degree of acidity, by which the iron was corroded, and a faint and scarcely perceptible blackness produced.

EXPERIMENT XL.

THREE or four drachms of *sal martis* were dissolved in half a pint of boiling water. After standing a few days, that the ochre might precipitate, the solution was passed through brown paper. The filtered liquor was perfectly clear, discovered no marks of acidity to the taste, and struck a deep black with the infusion of galls. In four or five days it let fall a very fine, light, yellow sediment, was again passed through the filter, and struck as before a deep black with the infusion of galls. I did not proſecute this experiment any further; being ſatisfied from the trial I had made, that the acid and the iron, the component parts of green vitriol, are not ſo eaſily ſeparated from each other as is commonly ſuppoſed. And it is probable that the acid, after the precipitation of the ochre, ſtill retains as much ferrugineous matter as is ſufficient to ſaturate it, when ſo much diluted with water.

EXPERIMENT XLI.

From a large copperas work eſtabliſhed near Wigan, I procured a quantity of the yellow ochre precipitated from green vitriol; and of a chocolate coloured pigment, made by expoſing the ochre to ſuch a degree of heat, as is ſufficient to ſeparate the acid, and give it what the painters term a BODY. Neither the ochre, nor the pigment were attracted by the magnet, a proof that they were both

both in a ſtate of calcination. Three grains of the ochre, and the ſame quantity of the chocolate coloured pigment were added to two glaſſes, each containing half an ounce of a decoction of the bark. The pigment communicated to the decoction its own peculiar colour; but the yellow ochre ſtruck with it a deep purpliſh black. Twenty drops of *ſp. c. c. vol.* made no change in the decoction with the pigment; but the other inſtantly loſt its black, and aſſumed a chocolate colour, exactly reſembling that of the pigment.

EXPERIMENT XLII.

THE reſult of the laſt experiment led me to imagine, that an alkali dropped upon the ochre would render it brown by abſtracting its acid; and on the contrary, that oil of vitriol added to the chocolate pigment would reſtore its yellow colour, and give it the property of ſtriking a black

black with vegetable aſtringents. I therefore diffuſed four grains of the ochre, and the ſame quantity of the pigment, in two glaſſes of water. To one I added twenty drops of *ſp. c. c. vol.* to the other the ſame quantity of *ol. vitriol.* The hartſhorn immediately precipitated the ochre in fine light flakes, but did not either efferveſce with it or alter its colour: The acid had no ſenſible effect on the pigment. Thus was I doubly diſappointed in the iſſue of this experiment.

EXPERIMENT XLIII.

A FEW drachms of the yellow ochre were well mixed with four ounces of ſpring water. As ſoon as the ochre ſubſided, the liquor above was carefully poured off, and paſſed through common filtering paper doubled. It had acquired a deep orange colour, was perfectly tranſparent, had an aluminous taſte, and was remarkably ſtyptic and aſtringent in the mouth.

mouth. A drachm of it ſtruck a deep green, inclining to black, with half an ounce of the bark decoction. I inſtilled twenty drops of *ſp. c. c. vol.* into a table ſpoonful of it: No effervesſcence enſued, but a very copious, flaky, and yellow ſediment was inſtantly produced. I kept the remainder of the orange coloured liquor, in an open glaſs veſſel for ſeveral weeks, without obſerving the leaſt ochery precipitation, or any diminution of its tranſparency. And this I apprehend is a proof, that a firm and laſting combination takes place, between certain proportions of the component parts of green vitriol.

THE ſame ochre was macerated in freſh parcels of water, till the filtered liquor had neither taſte, colour, nor the property of giving the leaſt black tinge to an infuſion of galls. The ochre was then dried by a very gentle heat, and two ſcruples of it were added to half an ounce of of the ſame decoction of the bark, which was uſed in the former experiments; but no change of colour enſued, only the decoction aſſumed a lighter yellow, whilſt the particles of the ochre floated in it.

EXPERIMENT XLIV.

SPIRIT of hartſhorn, dropped into a ſolution of green vitriol, occaſioned a copious precipitation, but no efferveſcence. It cannot be alledged therefore, that the yellow ochre contains no acid, becauſe it doth not raiſe a ſenſible ebullition with the volatile alkali.

THUS it appears that whatever deprives green vitriol of its acid, whether it be heat, the addition of an alkali, or repeated affuſions of water, deſtroys its power of ſtriking a black colour with vegetable aſtringents. May we not then juſtly conclude, that an acid is eſſentially neceſſary to this property, which it is more than

than probable depends upon the composition of the copperas as a mixt; and not upon either of its conſtituent parts ſeparately taken. Ink therefore is a combination of vitriolic acid, iron, and a certain proportion of vegetable aſtringent matter. (a) But as theſe principles bear but a weak relation to each other, their band of union is eaſily diſſolved, and it has long been a deſideratum in chemiſtry, to render it more fixed and permanent. Acids by attracting the aſtringent matter, with which it is evident from many of the foregoing experiments they have a ſtrong

(a) An ingenious friend of mine (Dr. Falconer of Bath) is of opinion that a double elective attraction takes place in the production of Ink. The acid forſakes the iron and combines with the vegetable aſtringent, ſeparating from it the phlogiſton, which unites with the iron. In ſupport of this hypotheſis he obſerves, 1. that mineral aſtringents, ſuch as earth of alum, &c. precipitate iron, as well as thoſe of the vegetable claſs; but affording no *phlogiſton*, the precipitate is in an ochrous ſtate. 2. That the black ſediment of ink is eaſily ſoluble in acids, whereas the *calces* precipitated by alkalis are of very difficult ſolution, owing to the almoſt entire loſs of their *phlogiſton*. For a perfect calx is found to be abſolutely inſoluble.

ſtrong affinity, diſcharge the black colour of ink. Alkalis on the contrary decompoſe it, by abſtracting the acid from the vitriol, and precipitating the iron. If the blackneſs hath been deſtroyed by an acid, the addition of an alkali in due proportion will reſtore it, and *vice verſa.* The reaſon why they thus counteract each others effects, is too obvious to require an explanation.

A RE-

A RECAPITULATION OF THE PRINCIPAL FACTS ASCERTAINED BY THE PRECEDING EXPERIMENTS.

1. THE PERUVIAN BARK, and many other vegetable bitters and aſtringents, yield their virtues as perfectly to cold as to boiling water.

2. As much of the Reſin of the Bark is diſſolved by cold maceration as by coction.

3. TRITURATION promotes and increaſes the ſolution of the Bark in water.

4. A STRONG infuſion of the Bark may, by means of triture, be prepared with great expedition.

5. QUICK

5. Quick lime neither quickens, nor increaſes the ſolution of the Bark in water.

6. The bark will not yield all its virtues either to cold water, boiling water, or rectified ſpirit of wine, nor probably to any other *menſtruum* ſingly employed. After thirty cold macerations, and twenty five coctions in different parcels of water, each *reſiduum*, though perfectly inſipid, yielded a bitter and aſtringent tincture, when digeſted in rectified ſpirit of wine. On the contrary after repeated digeſtions in rectified ſpirit of wine, when that *menſtruum* acquired neither taſte nor colour from the bark, cold water extracted from it a manifeſt degree of aſtringency.

7. Cold water is a more powerful ſolvent of the bark, than rectified ſpirit of wine. But brandy is a ſtronger *men-*

ſtruum

ſtruum than water, and Rheniſh wine than brandy.

8. The decoction, and infusion of the Peruvian Bark are very periſhable preparations.

9. Acids, bitters and astringents neutraliſe each other, forming what the chemiſts term a *tertium quid.* When combined together in due proportion, their taſte and ſmell is altered; the acids loſe the property of ſtriking a red colour with ſyrup of violets; and their antiſeptic powers in combination are double the ſum of them when ſeparately employed. The bark likewiſe, with vinegar, hath the property of reſtoring ſweetneſs to putrid ſubſtances, which Dr. Macbride affirms it hath not alone.

10. The vegetable acids combined with aſtringents, diminiſh their

aſtrictive power on the dead fibre; the mineral acids increaſe it.

11. ASTRINGENCY and BITTERNESS are diſtinct properties, and are united together in very different proportions in different vegetables.

12. NEITHER the taſte, nor the power of ſtriking a black colour with chalybeates, nor yet the property of hardening animal fibres, whether ſingly or collectively taken, are certain criteria of the aſtringent power of a medicine on the living body.

13. THE power of ſtriking a black colour with green vitriol is not always a teſt of aſtringency on the dead fibre; nor is it common to all vegetable aſtringents. Rue yields a faint black, on the addition of *ſal martis* to an infuſion of it, and yet is not aſtringent: Gentian on the contrary,

trary, ſtrikes no black, although it is a pretty ſtrong aſtringent.

14. PUTRID GALL is neutraliſed by all acids. But thoſe of the native vegetable claſs alone, entirely ſweeten it.

15. WHATEVER deprives green vitriol of its acid, whether it be heat, the addition of an alkali, or repeated affuſions of water, deſtroys its power of ſtriking a black colour with vegetable aſtringents.

16. AN ACID, contrary to the opinion of Dr. Lewis, appears to be eſſentially neceſſary to the above-mentioned property of green vitriol.

17. INK, ſeems to be a combination of vitriolic acid, iron, and a certain proportion of vegetable aſtringent matter.

ESSAY IV.

ON

THE USES

AND

OPERATION

OF

BLISTERS.

Certé hinc lucis aliquid erui poterit, quâ id tandem, in quo medicorum diligentiam deſidero, effici queat, ut accurata de veſicantium in diuturnis affectibus præcepta tradantur, quæ et perſpicuitatem habeant, et quaſdam errare in medendo non patientes vias.

FRIEND,

ESSAY IV.

ON THE USES, AND OPERATION OF BLISTERS.

THOUGH the action of cantharides as veſicatories was not unknown to the ancients, their application did not prevail much in practice, till the beginning of the laſt century. And as nothing hath tended more to enlarge the boundaries of ſcience, than the contentions of the learned; we owe perhaps, in a good meaſure, our preſent more accurate acquaintance with the virtues and operation of bliſters, to a diſpute amongſt the Italian phyſicians, relating to their uſe in a plague, which prevailed about the years 1575 and 1590. But although blisters are now almost universally employed, and experience hath ascertained their utility in various disorders; the theory of their action, as well as the mode of their operation, is yet undetermined, and remains a subject of litigation. Hence arises that diversity of opinions concerning the diseases in which they are indicated, the time of their application, and the parts to which they ought to be applied. Nor can we ever hope for uniformity in this particular amongst physicians, either with respect to their opinions or their practice, till a juster idea be formed of their mode of action, deduced from experience, and an attentive observation of their effects on the human body. When this is accomplished, a system of rules may be laid down for their right and advantageous application.

MEDICINES are generally divided into such

ſuch as act, 1. on the ſolids, 2. on the fluids: and Bliſters may be conſidered as belonging to each of theſe claſſes; though their relation is chiefly to the former. But here a queſtion occurs, whether veſicatories produce their effects by their external action on the body, or by the abſorption of their ſtimulating particles into the ſyſtem? Baglivy furniſhes us with two curious, though cruel experiments, of the injection of two ounces of the tincture of cantharides, into the jugular veins of a dog and a whelp. Great anxiety, violent pain, inſatiable thirſt, convulſions, and death, were the conſequences in each inſtance. But no certain or juſt inferences can be drawn from theſe experiments; becauſe medicines are not adminiſtered by injection into the blood veſſels; and ſubſtances much leſs acrid in their nature than cantharides, if conveyed directly and undiluted into the courſe of circulation, will be found to produce effects ſimilar, or at leaſt

leaſt equally deleterious. *(a)* When taken by the mouth in an over-doſe, the moſt dreadful ſymptoms ſucceed; an exulceration of the bladder and *urethra*, inflammation of the bowels, violent pains in the *hypogaſtrium*, extreme thirſt, a high fever attended with delirium, and at laſt death cloſes the melancholy ſcene. The like effects it is ſaid, though in a leſs degree, have been obſerved to ariſe from the application of bliſters. And it is upon theſe active powers of cantharides when abſorbed into the ſyſtem, properly modified and ſeaſonably applied, that the effects of veſicatories are ſuppoſed by ſeveral learned writers chiefly to depend. *(b)* The quicker contractions of the heart and arteries, in conſequence of their application in certain diſorders, they aſcribe,

(a) New milk injected into the veins of a dog proves a mortal poiſon.

Young on Opium, p. 6.

(b) Baglivy, Friend, Glaſs, Huxham, &c. &c.

aſcribe, not to a ſympathy with the ſkin, but to a ſtimulus circulated with the fluids, and acting immediately on the veſſels themſelves. And as Baglivy hath aſſerted that cantharides have the property of colliquating the blood, when mixed with it out of the body, they apprehend that the good effects of bliſters in fevers, attended with a glutinoſity and lentor in the fluids, ariſe principally, if not entirely, from their attenuating and diſſolving powers. But this theory of the operation of veſicatories is liable, I think, to many objections.

1. If their action depend upon the ſtimulus of the abſorbed cantharides, they ſhould in all caſes quicken the contractions of the vaſcular ſyſtem. But this is contradicted by experience; for in pleuriſies, peripneumonies, and other inflammatory diſeaſes, where the heart and arteries are already acting very ſtrongly,

ly, they abate the inflammation and lower the pulſe. (a)

2. The ſmall portion of cantharides, which may be carried into the courſe of circulation by the lymphatics of the ſkin, cannot I apprehend be adequate to the effects aſcribed to it, whether we conſider the large maſs of fluids with which it is mixed and diluted, or the coats of the veſſels lined with a mucus, which muſt defend them from any ſlight degree of acrimony. It may indeed be ſaid, that the uſual effects of a bliſter on the urinary paſſages ſhew, that the particles of cantharides are abſorbed in ſufficient quantity, to irritate and vellicate the internal parts of the body. But allowing this objection its full force, by granting what is diſputed by ſome, that the ſtrangury ariſes from the immediate action of the flies on the urinary paſſages, this

(a) Whytt's Experiments, Ph. Tranſact. Vol. 50, p. 2.

this by no means proves their ſtimulating power, when circulating with the general maſs of fluids. All extraneous bodies introduced into the blood, and not capable of being animalized, paſs off by one or other of the excretories. If they are of ſuch a nature as to be volatilized by the common heat of the body, they are eliminated by the lungs, and pores of the ſkin, along with the matter of inſenſible perſpiration. Garlick, onions, aſafætida, ſulphur, and moſt of the eſſential oils, afford examples of this kind. But if the extraneous matter be leſs volatile, if it be incapable of chemical mixture with the blood, or if it unite only with the ſerum, it will be carried to the kidneys, and paſs off by urine. Of this nature are cantharides; *(a)* and when their acrid particles are, in continual ſucceſſion, applied to

(a) BAGLIVY on mixing cantharides with the ſerum of the blood, found the powder precipitated ſoon after to the bottom of the veſſel, without having produced any change in the colour of that fluid.

to the highly ſenſible and nervous membrane, which lines the urinary ducts, can we wonder at the ſtrangury, and other painful effects which they produce. (a)

3. The ſame objection may be made to the attenuating power of cantharides, as introduced into the blood by means of bliſters. Is it at all probable, that a few grains of cantharides can act ſo powerfully, as to diſſolve a general lentor and viſcoſity of the whole maſs of fluids? Mercury it is true, in a very ſmall quantity, will excite a ſalivation: But it does not produce this effect, by breaking down the *craſis* of the blood, though the

(a) It is not improbable, that the nerves of the urinary paſſages are diſpoſed to be more irritated by the acrimony of the flies, than thoſe which are diſtributed to the other organs of the body. For Dr. Whytt hath ingeniouſly proved, that the different operation of medicines, depends very much on the particular nature, and diverſified ſenſibility, of the nerves of different parts of the body; by which they are differently affected by the ſame kind of ſtimulating ſubſtances.

Vid. Eſſay on Nerv. Diſ.

the continued uſe of it may have that tendency, but merely, as I conceive, by its partial ſtimulus on the ſalivary glands. An eminent practitioner informed me, that he had more than once ordered blood to be taken from patients under ſalivation, which he found not in a diſſolved, but even in a buffy ſtate. But it may be preſumed, I think, that cantharides are not poſſeſſed, in any conſiderable degree, of a colliquative power; for they have no chemical relation to the animal fluids, and Sir John Pringle hath proved, that they are by no means ſeptic. (a) As this, however, is a point of ſome importance, the two following experiments were repeated after Baglivy, in order to determine it.

EXPERIMENT I.

Four ounces of blood, juſt drawn from

(a) Append to Diſ. Army, Exp. 22.

from the arm, were divided into two equal portions; to one was added ten grains of *pulv. cantharid.* the other was kept as a ſtandard. The portion with cantharides coagulated at the ſame time with the ſtandard, and neither aſſumed a ſublivid, nor an aſh colour. Its ſurface was covered with a thin pellicle, but without the veſicles Baglivy deſcribes. After ſtanding a few hours, the craſſamentum in part diſſolved, as appeared from the colour of the ſerum, which was tinged with red; owing perhaps to a ſlight degree of agitation, which was uſed to mix the cantharides with the blood when freſh drawn.

The portion without the cantharides ſeparated into a clear, pale coloured ſerum, and a tough, aſh coloured craſſamentum; the ſurface of which contracted into the compaſs of a ſhilling, and retained that form till the putrefaction begun; which happened ſooner in the

the ſtandard, than in the other portion of blood.

EXPERIMENT II.

TEN grains of *pulv. cantharid.* added to two ounces of ſerum, tinged by the craſſamentum of a light, florid, crimſon colour, rendered it more liquid, and changed it to a dull red. Contrary to the aſſertion of Baglivy, it coagulated with great eaſe, and with leſs heat than an equal portion of the ſame ſerum without cantharides.

5. THE chief ſymptoms induced by bliſters, may be rationally accounted for, without having recourſe to the abſorption of the acrid particles, of which they are compoſed. Theſe ſymptoms are a quick pulſe, dryneſs of the tongue, thirſt, ſtrangury, &c. They quicken the pulſe in the low ſtate of fevers, by their ſtimulus on the ſkin, with which the whole

vascular system sympathises. They occasion thirst, dryness of the tongue, and an increase of fever, in the same way, viz. by their external irritation. But these effects ought to be ascribed to the improper and unseasonable use of blisters. When the inflammatory *diathesis* prevails universally, and strongly, without any partial obstruction, every stimulus must aggravate the symptoms; and blisters raised on the skin, by a cataplasm of mustard, or by the actual or potential cautery, where the irritation is confessedly external, would operate in the same manner as an epispastic of cantharides. But in cases where vesicatories are indicated, I have never found, on the strictest examination, the least increase of thirst, or dryness of the mouth, in consequence of their application. *(a)* The strangury

(a) The three histories which Baglivy relates of the effects of epispastics, carry very little authority with them; because the blisters were either ill timed, or laid on in too great

ſtrangury has by ſome been ſuppoſed to ariſe, not from an abſorption of cantharides, but from a ſympathy between the ſkin and the urinary paſſages. And it is urged, that a warm fomentation of milk

great numbers. The firſt caſe is that of a young man, of a bilious temperament, who after being heated, ſuddenly expoſed himſelf to the cold wind. He was ſeized with an *angina*, which terminated in a violent pleuriſy, attended with the ſtrongeſt ſymptoms of inflammation. Six veſicatories were applied at once, to different parts of his body; the conſequence of which was, a ſuppreſſion of the *ſputum*, tremors, convulſions, delirium, and death. The ſecond hiſtory is that of a cook, who was attacked with a convulſion of the lower jaw, which was ſoon after ſucceeded by ſpaſmodic contractions of the abdominal muſcles. The *pulvis cornachini* was preſcribed, and the next day four bliſters were applied. Vomiting, convulſive motions, and an oppreſſed breathing enſued. On the fourth day he died. This caſe was probably a locked jaw; a diſeaſe too frequently fatal. The third hiſtory is that of a young and ſlender woman, eight months advanced in pregnancy, who after ſuffering much pain was at length delivered. The pain however ſtill continued, accompanied with an uncommon tenſion of the belly. Four bliſters were applied at one and the ſame time, as in the former inſtances. The *lochia* were immediately ſuppreſſed, con-

and water applied to a bliſtered part, very quickly relieves this complaint, by removing or diminiſhing the irritation on the ſurface of the body. But I confeſs, the probability lies on the other ſide of the queſtion; and ſeveral reaſons incline me to think, that the ſtrangury is produced alone by the abſorption, and internal ſtimulus of the flies.

1. Neither muſtard, the actual or potential cautery, nor any other veſicating ſtimulus but cantharides, excite this complaint. And is it not ſtrange, that the

vulſions came on, and at laſt the poor patient fell a victim to death.

Baglivius de Veſicant. p. 70.

From the application of ſo many bliſters, it is not to be wondered at, that the thirſt, quickneſs of the pulſe, and other ſymptoms of acute diſeaſes were, according to the experience of Baglivy, greatly aggravated. Beſides, it is more than probable, that veſicatories are attended with greater inconveniences in warm, than in cold climates, becauſe the inhabitants of the former are generally of more irritable conſtitutions, and of more aduſt and bilious temperaments, than thoſe of the latter.

the urinary paſſages ſhould have ſuch a univerſal ſympathy with all the different parts of the body to which cantharides are applied, whilſt no ſuch conſent takes place, when any other veſicatory is made uſe of?

2. DRINKING plentifully prevents the ſtrangury; and ſurely it can produce this effect in no other way, than by diluting in the kidneys and bladder, the acrimonious particles of the flies.

3. A BLISTER laid upon the head immediately after ſhaving, is almoſt always ſucceeded by the ſtrangury; whereas no ſuch effect takes place, if the application be delayed twenty four hours. How are we to account for this fact, unleſs by ſuppoſing, that the ſubtiler parts of the cantharides enter more readily, and in greater quantity into the blood, after the ſcarf ſkin hath been removed by the razor? The effect of a

warm fomentation, in alleviating the troublesome symptoms of this complaint, arises partly, perhaps, from its sedative operation on the whole system, but chiefly, I imagine, from its washing off all those acrid particles adhering to the skin, which would otherwise enter into the blood, and increase, or at least continue the irritation in the urinary passages.

But although it be acknowledged, that the strangury is occasioned by the stimulus of the cantharides, acting internally, yet the explanation given above of this effect, removes, I think, every objection to what has been advanced. I shall proceed therefore to consider the operation of blisters, according to the division already laid down.

The diseases of the SOLIDA VIVA, in which they are indicated, are very numerous;

numerous; but taking a more general view of them, they may perhaps be reduced to three kinds.

1. WHERE THE ACTION OF THE MOVING FIBRES IS EITHER PARTIALLY, OR UNIVERSALLY TOO WEAK.

2. WHERE IT IS IRREGULAR.

3. WHERE IT IS PARTIALLY TOO STRONG.

IN the firſt caſe veſicatories are indicated, as a ſtimulus to the languid ſolids, to rouſe them to more vigorous contractions, to ſupport the *vis vitæ*, and to promote the ſalutary ſecretions. They tend to quicken the circulation, to raiſe the pulſe, and to animate the whole ſyſtem. Hence we may deduce their uſe and operation,

1. IN LOW NERVOUS FEVERS; when the

the ſpirits ſink, when the contractions of the heart grow languid, and the unhappy patient ſtruggles under anxiety, reſtleſſneſs, delirium, difficulty of breathing, and a load and oppreſſion about the *præcordia*. Theſe ſymptoms ariſe from debility, and denote a kind of nervous orgaſm, or ſpaſm on the vitals, which requires cordial medicines, aided by the application of bliſters. (a) An eminent practitioner hath indeed obſerved, that in theſe fevers, epiſpaſtics ſometimes aggravate all the ſymptoms, and by their irritation occaſion a ſmall and contracted pulſe. But this he aſcribes to a miſtake, either in the time, or place of their application. On the firſt ſigns of a delirium, when the urine turns pale, when the patient ſighs, is anxious, and becomes dull of hearing, or when his eyes ſparkle and look ſtaring, &c. he adviſes to cover the whole head with a bliſter. The

(a) *Vid.* Huxham on Fevers, p. 82.

The epiſpaſtic will thus be applied as near as poſſible to the part affected; and as the head is leſs ſenſible to the ſtimulus of cantharides, than any other part of the body, all the bad effects ariſing from too great irritation will be prevented. *(a)* Baglivy long ago remarked, that bliſters ſometimes excite a ſmall and contracted pulſe; and I apprehend in the claſs of diſeaſes now under conſideration, their utility muſt always be attended with a peculiar degree of uncertainty. This depends on the nature of theſe fevers, and the concomitant ſtate of the nerves. Whenever they are accompanied with little pain, but with a high degree of irritability, which is not unfrequently the caſe, bliſters, I think, will be found to be prejudicial, by increaſing the ſpaſm, and throwing the ſyſtem into confuſion. But if the body, however languid and enfeebled, has been accuſtomed through the

(a) Vid. Med. Eſſays of Edinburgh, Vol. 4. Art. 23.

the courſe of the diſeaſe, to the ſtimulus of pain, or if the nerves be not affected with an exceſs of ſympathetic ſenſibility, epiſpaſtics may be applied with ſafety and advantage.

2. IN the advanced ſtate of INFLAMMATORY FEVERS, when the patient becomes languid, or perhaps comatoſe, bliſters are highly ſerviceable. And they are found to be very efficacious in removing thoſe obſtinate and oppreſſive head-achs, which have reſiſted every previous evacuation, and which often continue to the laſt period of the diſtemper. (a) The ſame obſervation holds true in every other ſpecies of fever, where ſuch a train of ſymptoms occur as have been already deſcribed.

EVEN in malignant PETECHIAL FEVERS, notwithſtanding the great diſſolution

(a) *Vid.* Pringle's Diſ. of the Army, p. 134.

lution of the blood, and the ſuppoſed tendency of cantharides to increaſe that diſſolution, ſome of the moſt eminent practitioners have been bold enough to recommend bliſters. Thus Riverius ſays, *Ubi maxima eſt malignitas, unicum veſicatorium non ſufficit, ſed plura admovenda ſunt; ſoleo ego in magna morbi ſævitia, quinque locis admovere, cervici nimirum, utrique brachio, parti interiori inter cubitum et humerum, et utrique femori, parti etiam inferiori inter inguina et genua, cum felici ſucceſſu.* (a) Etmuller, treating of the ſame fevers aſſerts, *Si ulla eſt febris in qua veſicatoria conveniunt, eſt imprimis petechialis.* (b) And in the malignant, ulcerous ſore throat, it muſt be acknowledged that they are productive of the beſt effects. But with deference to theſe great authorities, I think bliſters ſhould be applied with the utmoſt caution, in all

(a) Riverii Opera, p. 541.
(b) Etmuller. Op. p. 365.

all cafes, attended with an highly putrid, and diffolved ftate of the fluids: For under fuch circumftances, they often exhauft the ftrength of the patient, by exciting an immoderate difcharge of bloody ferum; and they fometimes occafion a fudden, and fatal mortification.

3. In the small pox; when the patient is of a lax and weak habit, when the pulfe is low, feeble, and depreffed, and the fever infufficient for the expulfion and fuppuration of the puftules, epifpaftics are certainly indicated. *(a)* When the pocks are of the bloody kind, and attended with delirium, Dr. Mead affures us, that blifters may be ufed with equal fafety and advantage. And in this diftemper, whenever the maturation of the puftules does not regularly fucceed their eruption, and when anxiety, inquietude, difficulty of breathing,

(a) Hillary on the Small pox, p. 94. 95.

breathing, and delirium come on, the fever ſhould be quickened by warm cordial medicines, and eſpecially by the application of bliſters. (a) This is confirmed by the teſtimony of Dr. Tiſſot, in a late publication, who after pointing out the analogy between the action of opium and cantharides in the ſmall-pox, ſays, *Unicum eſt ſymptoma in quo dum hæc pulchra operantur à narcoticis caveo; ubi nimirum relicta cute, ad pulmonem acre devolvit viru, cum frequentiſſimo celerrimo, debilique pulſu, cutis ſiccitate, orthopnœa, anxietate, delirio. Gravis eſt ſanè caſus, et è peſſimis in medicina varioloſa, quem feliciter aliquoties, citò accerſitus, curavi, larga et accerima veſicatoria ſuris applicando, largiſſimos et calidos hauſtus decocti hordei, et ſambuci melliti preſcribendo, cum minimis doſibus ſulphuris aurati antimonii. Quatuor vel quinque lapſis horis, remittit frequentia pulſus, recedit*

(a) Mead, Sydenham, Morton.

recedit anxietas, madet cutis, increſcunt vires. Omnino liberato pectore, et demiſſa febre, juvari poteſt natura leni narcotico. Diu fluere crura juvat. (a) It is always accounted a bad ſymptom, when the ſewlling of the hands does not follow the tumour of the face, and the ſwelling of the feet that of the hands; and if the patient be threatened with this alarming circumſtance, epiſpaſtics ſhould be applied to the wriſts and ancles, a little before the inflammation of thoſe parts may be expected to begin. For they will not only tend to draw the humours thither, but will give them alſo a ſalutary vent. (b) When the fauces are covered with puſtules, and both deglutition and reſpiration are impeded by the ſwelling of the throat, bliſters applied to the neck are highly ſerviceable, as I have frequently

(a) Tiſſot. de Variolis, &c. *vid.* Sandifort. Theſaur. Vol. 2. p. 11.

(b) Huxham, p. 155.

frequently experienced. Dr. Tiſſot relates the hiſtory of a patient, under theſe circumſtances, who was ſuddenly relieved by the application of ſinapiſms to the feet. *Vidi hoc anno collum horride turgidum, educta è lecto ægra, et ſinapiſmis plantis pedum applicatis, intra viginti minuta, dimidiam diametri partem amiſiſſe. Horrendos verum eſt pedum patiebatur dolores, quos per bihorium tolerare ſuaſi; tunc tumentibus admodum cruribus, ſinapi removi; omnia pacabantur.* (a) In this inſtance, it is probable, that bliſters would have been no leſs efficacious than the ſinapiſms; and they would have been more eligible, becauſe productive of a leſs degree of pain and inflammation.

4. IN the APOPLEXY, whether ariſing from over diſtended veſſels, injuring the brain by preſſure, from the effuſion of blood within the *cranium*, or from a pituitous

(a) Sandifort's Theſaurus, Vol. 2. p. 16.

tuitous collection there; after attempting to relieve the head by bleeding, cupping the *occiput*, with deep ſcarifications, and uſing ſuch other evacuations, as the ſtate of the patient may require, bliſters may be applied, both to the head and extremities, with great advantage. By increaſing the circulation of the blood externally, and by producing a conſiderable diſcharge of ſerum, they will unload the veſſels of the brain; whilſt by their ſtimulus, they rouſe the torpid ſyſtem of nerves, excite the heart and arteries to quicker and more vigorous contractions, and thus powerfully contribute, to reſtore the equilibrium between the *vis motrix*, and *moles movenda*.

5. In the palsy. When this diſeaſe invades the whole body, bliſters are uſeful by their general ſtimulus. But they are moſt efficacious when the paralytic affection is not univerſal, but confined to ſome particular member or organ. Thus in

in palsies of the upper extremities, vesicatories applied to the *vertebræ* of the neck, and going obliquely to the shoulder, are remarkably useful. And when the disease attacks the lower extremities, they are equally efficacious, when laid upon the region of the *os sacrum*. In both cases, experience demonstrates that blisters thus applied are much more efficacious, than when laid upon the extremities themselves. As most of the nerves which go to the bladder, pass through the *foramina* of the *os sacrum*, vesicatories have been very successfully applied to that region, for the cure of an incontinence of urine. And it is probable, that they would be much more certain and powerful in their operation, if a proper attention was paid, in their external application, to the origin and course of the nerves. (a)

6. IN the GUTTA SERENA, when it proceeds

(a) *Vid.* Lond. Medical Observ. Vol. 2. p. 318.

proceeds from a paralytic affection of the retina, bliſters applied to the forepart of the head, ſo as to cover the nerves which iſſue through the *ſupra* orbital *foramina*, and ſpread themſelves on the forehead, are highly ſerviceable, as I have more than once experienced.

7. IN the TYMPANITES, Celſus adviſes to make ulcers in ſeveral parts of the belly, and to keep them running. But we are furniſhed by means of epiſpaſtics, with a much more effectual, as well as more humane remedy. Dr. Mead recommends their application in this diſorder; and it is probable they may do ſervice, both as ſtimulants and antiſpaſmodics, except where the caſe is complicated with a mortification of the bowels.

8. IN the RICKETS, Boerhaave recommends bliſters, to ſtimulate the languid veſſels, and reſolve the mucous concretions.

9. IN

9. In schirrous tumours of the conglobate glands of the neck, bliſters applied to the head, or behind the ears, have a good effect. The finer parts of the cantharides, being abſorbed by the lymphatics, are carried immediately to the obſtructed glands, and by their ſtimulus tend to diſcuſs thoſe indolent ſwellings. A young lady who had a hard, glandular tumour in her neck, which ſucceeded the ſmall-pox, and had reſiſted very powerful applications, was lately cured of it by the application of a bliſter behind her ear, which I directed on account of an inflammation in one of her eyes. If the tumour be ſeated in the inguinal glands, veſicatories ſhould be applied to the thighs. In ſuch caſes I have laid bliſters over the glands themſelves, but without any beneficial effect.

10. In thoſe ſchirrous, or œdematous tumours of the joints, uſually called white swellings, which after a tedious and ill conditioned ſuppuration,

corrupt the *synovia*, shorten the tendons, make the bones carious, and destroy the articulation, blisters applied to the part affected, have been sometimes highly serviceable. *(a)* But their operation should be assisted by the internal use of the Peruvian bark, calomel, or other alterative and deobstruent medicines. *(b)*

OTHER diseases, arising from the too weak action of the solids, might be enumerated; but sufficient has been said to prove the efficacy and utility of blisters in such cases.

2. WHERE THE ACTION OF THE MOVING FIBRES IS IRREGULAR, vesicatories are indicated, both as stimulants and antispasmodics.

CONVULSIVE

(a) Vid. Medical Transactions, Vol. 1. p. 104.

(b) THE Abbe Chappe mentions an epidemic disease in Russia, probably a species of the bronchocele, which the natives cure by the application of tobacco and sal ammoniac well masticated. The tumours are of the size of an apple, they rise suddenly, and if neglected soon become incurable.

Travels into Siberia, p. 353.

Convulsive motions or spasms ſeem generally to ariſe from ſome peculiar irritation of the nervous ſyſtem. And whether the brain be originally, or only ſympathetically affected, whatever rouſes and engages the attention of the mind, will ſeldom fail to afford relief, by leſſening, or deſtroying the ſenſe of that irritation. Bliſters therefore are indicated in ſuch diſeaſes, to ſtimulate and excite pain in a part of the body that is ſound. For according to the aphoriſm of Hippocrates, *Duobus doloribus ſimul obortis, non in eodem loco, vehementior obſcurat alterum.* (a) Dr. Whytt relates the caſe of a patient, who had an alternate motion of the muſcles of the *abdomen*, which was cured by a circular bliſter, of about eight inches diameter, applied to the part affected. (b) The ſame author acquaints us, that where epilepſies take their riſe from an uneaſy

 ſenſation

(a) Lib. 2. Aph. 46.

(b) Whytt on Nerv. Diſ. p. 460.

ſenſation in ſome part of the arm or leg, he has found veſicatories, applied to thoſe parts, the moſt effectual remedies. (a)

In the convulſions which ſometimes precede the eruption of the ſmall-pox, bliſters act as powerful antiſpaſmodics. But they ſhould not, upon ſlight occaſions, be employed in this ſtate of the diſeaſe, leſt by their ſtimulus they aggravate the fever, and increaſe the number of puſtules. When ſuch ſymptoms occur in the ingrafted ſmall-pox, as indicate the uſe of veſicatories, it is ſaid that they will ſucceed the beſt, if applied to the arms, over the part where the variolous matter was inſerted. This I am informed is the preſent practice of an ingenious phyſician, and celebrated inoculator, who merits all the honours which have been conferred upon him, by one of the wiſeſt potentates in Europe.

In

(a) Whytt on Nerv. Diſ. p. 461.

In the idiopathic Epilepſy, the application of veſicatories to the head is recommended by Hoffman, Riverius, Piſo, and Mead; who ſupport their recommendation, by many authentic caſes and hiſtories. Celſus mentions ſeveral remedies for the epilepſy, which are very ſingular; ſuch as drinking the warm blood of a gladiator juſt ſlain, eating human or horſes fleſh, or the parts of generation of certain animals. If theſe things had any efficacy, it muſt ariſe from the repugnancy of nature to them, and from the ſtrong and painful ſenſations of mind, which ſuch ſhocking and diſguſting remedies could not fail to excite. Upon the ſame principle, Boerhaave cured the epileptics in the poor houſe at Haerlem. *(a)*

Hoffman relates that he has found epiſpaſtics of excellent uſe in the ſpaſmodic aſthma; *(b)* and Dr. Whytt confirms the

(a) See the Account in Kaw Boerhaave.

(b) Hoffman de Veſicant.

the teſtimony of Hoffman by his own experience. *(a)*

In fixed pains of the bowels from ſpaſms, though there are no evident marks of inflammation, the application of bliſters to the *abdomen* may be recommended. Sir John Pringle aſſures us, that he has oftener than once ſeen a patient relieved in his bowels, as ſoon as he felt the burning of his ſkin; and at the ſame time have ſtools by a purge, or a clyſter, which had not operated before. In ſevere, and continued vomitings, when the ſtomach is affected with very painful convulſive motions, I have obſerved the moſt ſalutary effects from the application of a veſicatory to the epigaſtric region. Hence we may conclude, that bliſters act

(a) Nerv. Diſ. p. 495. Epiſpaſtics have alſo been found to be very ſerviceable in the *tuſſis convulſiva*. *Vid.* Ridley's Obſerv. p. 91.

act not in ſuch caſes as evacuants, but as antiſpaſmodics.

3. When the action of the solida viva is too strong.

It is yet a ſubject of diſpute amongſt phyſicians, whether epiſpaſtics are uſeful, or detrimental in inflammatory fevers. Hoffman bears the ſtrongeſt teſtimony againſt their application in ſuch caſes; *(a)* and Baglivy from his own experience aſſerts, "*Quod delirantibus cum febre acuta, lingua arida, et indicijs magnæ viſcerum inflammationis, ſi applicentur veſicantia, omnia in pejus ruunt, et magna ex parte moriuntur convulſi.*" *(b)* Alpinus ſays, *Nunquam probare potui, in acutis febribus, veſicantium uſum, quod calorem febrilem augeant, vigilias doloremque concitent, et deliria inducant, coctionem impediant, non minus*

(a) De Veſicant. uſu. §. 17.

(b) Praxis. p. 102.

minus et motui humorum critico obſint, quum incertus ſit locus ad quem, vel per quem criſis eſt futura." (a) Sir John Pringle acquaints us, that his firſt practice in every inflammatory fever was to bliſter; but afterwards, when he found that a ſolution of the fever was not to be procured by ſuch means, he confined the uſe of epiſpaſtics to thoſe ſtates of the diſeaſe, in which he could be moſt aſſured of their efficacy. (b) Huxham, if I miſtake not, obſerves that to bliſter in the beginning of inflammatory fevers is to add fuel to the fire; and Dr. Whytt expreſſly ſays, that in fevers, where there is no partial obſtruction, or inflammation, veſicatories are of little ſervice, and are ſometimes

(a) Medicin. Method. lib. 5. p. 173.

(b) In the ſecond ſtage of the jail or hoſpital fever, when the pulſe is quick and full, Sir John Pringle hath uſed bliſters, but without ſucceſs. Nay upon the firſt attack, the whole head has been bliſtered, and the oozing kept up for ſome days, without relieving it, or preventing any of the uſual ſymptoms.

Diſ. of the Army, p. 318.

ſometimes hurtful; unleſs perhaps towards the end of the diſeaſe, when the pulſe begins to ſink. *(a)*

On the other hand Sydenham, whoſe authority muſt have great weight, from his accurate attention to the *juvantia* and *lædentia* in all diſeaſes, adopted the uſe of bliſters in the continued acute fever, which prevailed in the years 1673, 1674, 1675. The ſymptoms of this fever, as he deſcribes them, indicate a very high degree of inflammation; and his practice was, firſt to take away a ſufficient quantity of blood from the arm, and then to apply a large epiſpaſtic to the neck: At the ſame time he employed the cooling regimen. Dr. Friend ſays, that in acute fevers, the ſafeſt and moſt ſpeedy relief is afforded by veſicatories. Nor are we to be too ſcrupulous about accomodating them to the conſtitution, or ſtate of the patient;

(a) Philoſ. Tranſ. Vol. 50. pt. 2. p. 578.

patient; for whatever his habit of body may be, if the fever rages beyond measure, the slight inconvenience of a blister is rather to be endured, than the life of the patient endangered; for in these cases, the only hope is in blisters. They derive the febrile matter from the brain, and assist and promote the other discharges, those especially by sweat and urine. (a) Dr. Glass also, in his learned commentaries, recommends the application of blisters in inflammatory fevers. "*In febribus inflammatoriis, post debitam sanguinis missionem, locum habet id remedij; atque licet motus arteriarum, etiamnum nimis veloces, ab eo intendantur, brevi tantum intervallo id fiet, postea quidem, eliquatis densis humoribus, pulsus sentientur molliores, et febres erunt leniores.*" (b) "I have more than once in an evening," says Dr. Lind in his valuable paper on fevers

(a) *Vid.* Friend de Vesicant.

(b) Glass Comment. p. 235.

fevers and infection, "ordered eight or ten patients to be blistered, and have left them with a quick pulse, great heat, immoderate thirst, a pain, confusion, and heaviness of the head, and what to a physician conversant with such fevers, communicates a most certain knowledge of the condition of the patient, such a lifeless, sunk state of the eyes, as denoted great danger. But the next morning I found these patients with a lively, brisk eye, a calm pulse, and with a desire to get out of bed. (a) Other authorities to the same purpose might be advanced.

How then are we to determine this dispute? May not the truth in this, as in most other litigated points, lie in the middle way between the opposite opinions? If so, the following conclusion may perhaps be justified: That whenever the inflammatory *diathesis* prevails strongly, and

(a) Lind on Fevers and Infection, p. 9.

and uniformly throughout the ſyſtem, and no one part is more affected than the reſt, veſicatories are pernicious and detrimental. But when peculiar ſymptoms of inflammation attack the head, the lungs, &c. and prevail more in thoſe parts, than the reſt of the body, bliſters are indicated, and often prove remarkably uſeful. And in ſuch caſes they are found from experience, to leſſen the impetus of the blood upon the veſſels of the inflamed part, to abate the fever and heat of the body, and to diminiſh very remarkably the quickneſs of the pulſe. *(a)* Whatever may

(a) To underſtand more clearly the action of bliſters in ſuch caſes, it is neceſſary to form a juſt idea of the nature of inflammation, which ſeems to conſiſt in an increaſed alternate contraction of the veſſels of the part affected. If the inflammation be large, or the part inflamed very ſenſible, the whole nervous ſyſtem will be ſo affected by the pain, as to render the heart and larger arteries more irritable; and the force of the circulation will, of courſe, be greatly increaſed through the whole body. This ſtate is what is called the inflammatory *diatheſis*. In the cure of

may have been the original cauſe of a fever, it will be continued, and often greatly increaſed, by any particular inflammation, which may happen to have taken riſe from it. Under theſe circumſtances, the application of a bliſter to a neighbouring part, will ſometimes produce a reſolution of the diſeaſe, by leſſening the impetus of the fluids on the inflamed part, by making a conſiderable derivation of ſerous humours from it, and

of inflammation therefore, two indications are to be attended to; 1. to diminiſh the force of the circulation in general; 2. to abate the action of the veſſels in the part affected. The former is to be attempted by venæſection, and the antiphlogiſtic regimen; the latter by emollient and ſedative applications, and frequently by bliſtering the neighbouring parts. For the impetus of the fluids, in the veſſels of the part to which the veſicatory is applied, is much more augmented in proportion, than the force of the circulation in general. And as there ſeems to be only a certain degree of nervous energy, exerted in the body at one time, the increaſe of its action in one part, will neceſſarilly diminiſh it in another. And thus the original inflammation is cured, by exciting another contiguous to it.

and by rendering the mind leſs ſenſible of the painful irritation, which excites and continues the inflammation. Upon theſe principles, I apprehend, we may eaſily explain the action, and deduce from them the uſes of epiſpaſtics in the following diſeaſes.

1. In the SYMPTOMATIC PHRENITIS or DELIRIUM, which accedes indifferently to the bilious, malignant, or inflammatory fever. If the lowneſs of the pulſe admits not of venæſection, the cure muſt be atttempted by leeches and bliſters.(a) On this ſubject, Dr. Whytt furniſhes us with a practical obſervation of importance: that in fevers, where the ſubſtance of the brain is affected, and not its membranes, he has never found any benefit from the uſe of bliſters. And he always ſuſpects the brain to be affected, when a fever and delirium come on, without

(a) *Vid.* Pringle on the Diſ. of the Army, p. 138.

without any preceding head ach, or redneſs in the *tunica albuginea* of the eyes. This kind of fever he has met with ſeveral times, and has obſerved it to be generally fatal. *(a)* But I have lately had under my care a patient, whoſe caſe furniſhes an exception to this valuable obſervation; and as there is ſomething ſingular and curious in it, it may not perhaps be an uſeleſs digreſſion, to give a detail of the moſt intereſting circumſtances which attended it.

M. B. a maid ſervant, aged twenty four, being with child, was turned out of her place, and obliged to go into the poor houſe, where ſhe remained ſeveral weeks after her delivery. But ſunk with low diet, oppreſſed with uneaſineſs, and exhauſted with nurſing, ſhe was taken back by her friends, who were aſſiſted in their endeavours to recruit and reſtore her

Q ſtrength,

(a) Vid. Phil. Tranſ. Vol. 50. pt. 2. p. 578.

ſtrength, by the charitable benefactions of a neighbouring gentlewoman, diſtinguiſhed for her humanity. Auguſt 12th. 1766, a few days after her return home, ſhe was ſeized with a fever, which begun with a coldneſs and ſhivering, and was ſucceeded by heat. On the 18th I ſaw her, and found her in a delirium, with a low and feeble pulſe. Her eyes were ſunk, but without the leaſt redneſs or inflammation, nor had ſhe complained of any preceding pain in the head. Her urine was ſometimes pale, ſometimes high coloured. Her ſkin had that kind of heat, which is not eaſily deſcribed, but which leaves a diſagreeable ſenſation in the hand that feels it. Her tongue was dry and blackiſh; ſhe had a fluſhing every now and then in her face, and her belly was immoderately looſe; and to all theſe complaints an almoſt total deafneſs was added. In the afternoon there was generally a ſlight remiſſion of the ſymptoms.

A LARGE

A LARGE bliſter was ordered to be laid betwixt her ſhoulders, and a cordial, diaphoretic, and lightly aſtringent mixture was preſcribed.

AUG. 20. The delirium ceaſed. Her pulſe and heat were natural, her looſeneſs was abated, but her deafneſs ſtill continued. Two bliſters were directed to be applied behind her ears.

21. THERE ſeemed to be no appearance of fever; and the deafneſs was going off, though the bliſters had not been applied. She complained of a numbneſs in her right leg, which on examination I found to be cold and motionleſs. Directions were given to rub it well with the fleſh bruſh, and a large cataplaſm of muſtard and oat meal *ana p. æ.* was ordered to be applied to her foot.

24th. THE palſy was almoſt removed.

In other reſpects ſhe was well, except the pain occaſioned by the cataplaſm.

30th. SHE had the perfect uſe of her leg.

SEPTEMB. 3d. Though the inflammation occaſioned by the cataplaſm was very inconſiderable, yet ſhe complained of great pain ariſing from it. Her foot was therefore fomented with a decoction of chamomile and poppy heads, to which a ſufficient quantity of milk was added; and afterwards a white bread poultice was applied to it.

5th. THIS morning ſhe was ſeized with convulſions of the epileptic kind, and had ſix fits ſucceſſively. She was cold, feeble and languid, and complained much of ſickneſs and pain in her head. The following medicines were preſcribed.

℞. *Tinct.*

℞. *Tinct. valerian. volat. tinct. fuliginis, ana* ℥ſs. *laud. liquid. gutt.* xl. *m. cap. cochl. parv.* ij. *omni hora, ex cyatho aquæ ſpirituſque vini gallici.*

℞. *Rad. valerian. ſylveſt.* ℥ſs. *aq. fontan.* ℥xij. *coque parum, et adde aſafœtid.* ʒiſs. *m. f. enema ſtatim injiciend.*

6th. SHE was better, and had no return of the fits; but complained ſtill of violent pain in the foot.

7th. SHE continued free from the fits. Her head was eaſier, but her foot was ſtill painful. Yeſterday in the afternoon, ſhe was ſuddenly deprived of her ſight, without the leaſt previous pain or uneaſineſs in her eyes. No inflammation, opacity, or alteration of any kind appeared externally; except that the pupils were more than ordinarily dilated. On holding a lighted candle cloſe to her eye, the pupil did not con-

 tract

tract itſelf, and ſhe had not the leaſt perception of the light. As I apprehended her blindneſs to be a *gutta ſerena*, ariſing from a paralytic affection of the retina, I ordered her forehead to be frequently rubbed with the *liniment. volatile*, made with equal quantities of *ol. oliv.* and *ſp. ſalis ammon. cum calce viva*; and afterwards a flannel, moiſtened with the mixture, to be left upon the part. It was hoped that by this ſtimulus, applied immediately to the nerves which iſſue from the eyes, through the *ſupra* orbital *foramina*, the retina might be reſtored to its proper ſenſibility. And the event in ſome meaſure anſwered my expectations; for before night, ſhe was able to diſtinguiſh the light of a candle. But the recovery of her ſight was both imperfect, and of ſhort continuance.

8th. SHE was ſtill blind, and more ſtupid and heavy than uſual. She was frequently ſick, and vomited her food, but

but refused all medicines. A blister was ordered to be applied to her forehead.

9th. SHE had perfectly recovered her sight. No sooner did the blister begin to operate, but she had a glimmering of light, the pain occasioned a flow of tears, and she was gradually, during the action of the vesicatory, restored to the use of her eyes.

10th. SHE still retained the perfect use of her eyes; was more chearful and lively, had no pain in her head, and complained less of her foot. As she seemed to be in a fair way of recovering her former state of health, I left her, after giving the proper directions with respect to her diet.

N. B. THE young woman continued to recover, and about ten days afterwards I saw her perfectly well.

2. IN OPTHALMIAS. Inflammations of the eyes are frequently cured, by making a derivation from the part affected, either by means of leeches, or of bliſters. Perhaps both might be uſefully applied at the ſame time; the leeches near the external angle of the eye, and the bliſters behind the ears; or according to the preſent more efficacious method of practice, upon the forepart of the head. To conſpire with their operation, if the flux of humours to the eyes be great, a briſk purge may be adminiſtered, to make a revulſion. And thus, I apprehend, a cure may be compleated, without draining the whole body by large and repeated venæſections. Hoffman diſſuades us from applying epiſpaſtics to the neck in opthalmias. "*In opthalmia egregij ſunt uſus; ſed obſervavi, quod in nucha non adeo conducant, ſed potius dolor inde augeatur; quum contra pedibus admota, ſæpe ſimulac*

ſimulac humor ſtillare incipit, dolorem levent." (a)

3. IN NASAL HÆMORRHAGES, bliſters applied to the back have been ſerviceable; (b) and may we not from analogy conclude, that they would be equally uſeful in HÆMOPTOES?

4. IN the INFLAMMATORY ANGINA, Sydenham recommends the application of a large, and ſtrong epiſpaſtic between the ſhoulders, having premiſed bleeding and purging. Sir John Pringle mentions another remedy, whoſe mode of operation ſeems to be ſimilar to that of bliſters; viz. the application of a piece of flannel to the throat, moiſtened with two parts of *ol. oliv.* and one of *ſp. c. c. vol.* or in ſuch a proportion as the ſkin will bear. By this means the neck, and ſometimes

(a) De Veſicant. uſu. §. 12.
(b) Cullen's Clinical Lect.

ſometimes the whole body is put into a ſweat. But I imagine it is not by the *diaphoreſis*, ſo much as by the revulſion which it produces, that this application is ſo efficacious: And upon this principle, perhaps a bliſter would be ſtill more ſerviceable. Its operation indeed would not be ſo quick; but the copious derivation of ſerous humours, from veſſels nearly connected with the inflamed parts, would much more than balance the comparative ſlowneſs of its operation. *(a)*

5. In the firſt ſtage of the ANGINA MALIGNA, a bliſter applied to the nape of the neck, or to each ſide of the throat, produces very ſalutary effects. But as the ſkin in this diſeaſe is particularly diſpoſed

(a) On looking into the laſt Edit. of Sir John Pringle's Diſeaſes of the Army, I find a note in which he informs us, that in later practice, beſides a bliſter to the back, in bad caſes he lays one acroſs the throat: at other times he has applied ſeven or eight leeches under the *fauces*, p. 173.

diſpoſed to inflammation, I have ſeen inconveniences ariſe from the too powerful ſtimulus of the cantharides. Of late therefore, I have directed the *emplaſt. veſicatorium*, of the London Diſpenſatory, to be mixed with an equal, or double proportion of the *emplaſt. ſtomachicum*, and to this compoſition, have added a drachm or two of camphor, properly comminuted with rectified ſpirit of wine. Such a plaiſter I have repeatedly experienced to be ſufficiently efficacious as a bliſter; and the antiſeptic ingredients it contains, coincide with the general indication of correcting putrefaction.

If a bliſter plaiſter, after being moderately warmed before the fire, be covered with a fine, ſoft piece of muſlin, it will occaſion much leſs irritation, produce no ſtrangury, or but in a ſlight degree, and, when to be removed, will ſeparate from the ſkin, with great facility: Nor will ſuch a covering prevent its veſicating effects,

effects. Hence bliſters may in this manner, be applied with advantage, whenever the ſkin is diſpoſed to eryſipelatous inflammation from its extreme ſenſibility; or when their evacuating powers are wanted, with a diminution of their ſtimulus. In puerperal caſes alſo, they may thus be uſed, without danger of inflaming the *uterus*, by their action on the urinary paſſages.

6. In a true PERIPUEUMONY, eſpecially when the inflammation is great, repeated bleeding is the principal remedy; and Dr. Whytt diſſuades us from the early application of bliſters. But when the diſeaſe is of a mixed kind, when the lungs are not ſo much inflamed, as loaded with a pituitous matter, when bleeding gives but little relief, when the pulſe though quick is ſmall, when the patient is not able to bear evacuations, and the diſeaſe hath continued for ſome time, in ſuch circumſtances epiſpaſtics will produce

duce remarkably good effects. *(a)* Sir John Pringle says that a pleurisy, taken in the beginning, may often be cured by one large bleeding, and a blister laid to the side affected. If there be no particular stitch, but only a general oppression, the vesicatory may be applied to the back, and afterwards if the disease be obstinate, first to one side and then to the other. Whether applied to the chest, or to the extremities, it will relieve the breast, promote expectoration, and lower the pulse. In pulmonic disorders, Huxham recommends blistering the legs; and he observes that when they ulcerate the extremities severely, they commonly give great relief. *(b)*

7. IN the CHRONIC ASTHMA, when the patients strength is very much reduced,

(a) Phil. Trans. Vol. 50. pt. 2.

(b) *Vid.* Essay on Fevers, p. 219. and Obs. de Aere. et Morb. Epid. Vol. 2.

ced, bliſters are highly efficacious. But they ſhould never be applied to the cheſt, when the *dyſpnoea* is very ſevere; becauſe they render the motion of the intercoſtal muſcles more difficult and painful, as well as obſtruct reſpiration by their preſſure and tenacity. In theſe caſes volatiles are highly uſeful.

8th. In the SMALL POX, when it is attended with rawneſs, ſoreneſs, and great heat in the mouth and throat, and a ſharp rheum or ſtoppage in the noſtrils, bliſters are found to be very ſucceſsful. And in this diſeaſe, whenever the *membrana ſchneideriana* is affected, a revulſion from it is indicated; otherwiſe towards the cloſe of it, the patient will be in danger of ſuffocation. (a)

9th. In COUGHS, attended with fever, pain

(a) *Vid.* Eſſay on Fevers, p. 219. and Obſ. de Aere. et Morb. Epid. Vol. 2. p. 140, 149.

pain in the ſide, and a pituitous infarction of the lungs, bliſters are highly efficacious, in abating the fever, lowering the pulſe, and removing the inflammatory obſtruction. This Dr. Whytt hath ſatiſfactorily proved, by a detail of caſes, laid before the Royal Society, and publiſhed in the Philoſ. Tranſ. vol. 50.

10th. In the INFLAMMATION OF THE LIVER, one of the beſt remedies is a large bliſter laid over the part affected. (a)

11th. In the INFLAMMATION of the STOMACH and INTESTINES, in the ILEUS and INFLAMMATORY COLICK, epiſpaſtics are found to be ſerviceable. (b)

12th. In the DYSENTERY, when the pains in the belly are too fixed to yield to fomenta-

(a) Pringle's Diſ. of the Army, p. 151.
(b) Ibid.

fomentations, they are relieved by a blister, applied to the *abdomen*. *(a)*

13th. Blisters are remarkably serviceable in the DIARRHOEA, which sometimes attends the MEASLES; probably because they lessen the inflammation, which in this disease falls on the intestines.

14th. In the RHEUMATISM, SCIATICA, and GOUT, Hoffman commends the use of vesicatories, because they set in motion, and evacuate the supposed acrid matter, which is impacted in the nervous and tendinous parts. Pringle advises their application to the part affected, in the rheumatism and sciatica; and a celebrated Professor at Edinburgh asserts, that they seldom fail of success in the rheumatism, when applied before a swelling of the part comes on. *(b)* Huxham also bears testimony

(a) Pringle's Dis. of the Army, p. 202.
(b) Cullen's Clinical Lectures.

teſtimony in favour of epiſpaſtics: "*In crudeliſſimo rheumatiſmo, nihil magis prodeſt quam veſicatoria, inter ſcapulas ſuperimpoſita.* (*a*)

THUS much for the action of bliſters on the MOVING FIBRES. Their operation on the FLUIDS, depends upon their medicinal powers as attenuants, and evacuants; and theſe, perhaps, ariſe ſolely from their ſtimulus on the ſolids. By quickening the alternative contractions of the veſſels, they prevent the ſtagnation of the juices; hence their attenuating effects: and by exciting an inflammation externally, they occaſion a flux of humours to the ſkin, and a conſequent evacuation of them. It ſeems therefore to be almoſt unneceſſary, to conſider veſicatories as belonging to this ſecond claſs of medicines. But as ſome intereſting particulars, relating to their operation as evacuants, have

 been

(*a*) De Colico Damnoniorum.

been omitted in the preceding part of this attempt to investigate their uses, I shall briefly consider them under this head.

1. IN NERVOUS FEVERS, blisters act not only as a stimulus, but as a drain; and they should not be too soon dried up. Huxham says the more they discharge, and the better it is for the patient: and when the first blisters heal up, he recommends the application of others.

2. In DROPSIES, particularly in the *anasarca*, blisters applied to the legs produce a very copious discharge of serous humours, but they should be used with caution, because they sometimes occasion a spreading, painful, and dangerous inflammation. I was lately witness to a fatal case of this kind. The patient laboured under a dropsy of the *thorax*, and a general *anasarca*. His legs and thighs were swoln to an amazing size.

Vesica-

Veſicatories were applied to the extremities, a little above each ankle, and by unloading the cellular membrane they at firſt afforded great relief, but in a few days an eryſipelas enſued, which extended itſelf over the whole legs and part of the thighs, producing ſuch excruciating pain, that the patient, whoſe ſtrength had been before nearly exhauſted, ſunk under the anguiſh. — Whenever it is thought expedient to employ bliſters, for the removal of anaſarcous ſwellings, they ſhould be covered with fine, ſoft muſlin, in the manner before deſcribed.

3. In the LYMPHATIC or CRYSTALLINE SMALL POX, veſicatories are recommended as evacuants, both by Huxham and Mead. For by the ſeaſonable diſcharge of the ſeroſities, the fever, which increaſes when there is no further derivation of humours to the ſkin, is happily moderated, if not prevented.

4. In the WARTY SMALL POX, bliſters

are very uſeful evacuants; becauſe the matter being too thick, can neither ſuppurate, nor paſs off by urine. *(a)*

5. IN the CONVULSIONS to which children are ſubject the beſt practical writers adviſe the application of bliſters, chiefly on account of the drain which they produce. The plenty of nutrition which nature hath provided for the young animal, from the time of its birth, neceſſarily creates many redundancies, which in a healthy ſtate, are carried off by the glands of the ſkin, by urine, or by ſtool. Hence when the infant is arrived to a certain growth, an eruption, called the red gum, uſually appears on the ſurface of the body, and frequently at the ſame time, there is a diſcharge from the glands behind the ears, and in the groin. During theſe excretions, the child for the moſt part is lively and well; but as the equilibrium of

(a) Vid. Mead de Variolis.

of health, in ſuch delicate ſubjects, is eaſily diſturbed, their continuance is very precarious. And if ſome new evacuation, be not ſubſtituted in the room of them, diſeaſe will unavoidably enſue. For ſo exquiſite is the ſenſibility of the nervous ſyſtem in children, that a very ſlight degree of irritation will, in their tender bodies, excite convulſions. In ſuch circumſtances, the utility of bliſters is obvious, and might be inferred even *à priori*, if experience had not given a ſanction to their application. But their good effects are warranted by the moſt undoubted teſtimonies. And as a proof how ſalutary it is, to promote the diſcharge of the ſuperabundant juices in children, Willis relates the caſe of a girl, who was ſubject to the epilepſy, and in one of her fits fell into the fire, and burnt her face and forehead in the moſt ſhocking manner. The accident however was attended with this good effect, that as long as the ulcers remained open,

open, ſhe was free from the diſorder. Hollerius furniſhes us with a ſimilar example. A girl had from her infancy a running ſore in her head: It was ſuddenly healed up, and ſhe became epileptic. Variety of remedies were tried to no purpoſe: Duretus was conſulted, who recommended the application of beet leaves to her head, which brought on a large diſcharge, and removed her epilepſy. *(a)* Agreeable to this is the obſervation of Hippocrates, that running ſores of the head happening to children, prevent the convulſions. "*Quibuscunque quidem pueris exiſtentibus, erumpunt ulcera in caput, et in aures, aç in reliquum corpus; et qui ſalivoſi fiunt, ac mucoſi, hi ipſi in progreſſu ætatis facillimè degunt: Qui vero mundi ſunt, et neque ulcus ullum, neque mucus, neque ulla ſaliva prodit, neque in uteris purgationem fecerunt, talibus periculum imminet, ut ab hoc morbo (i. e. epilepſia) corripi-*

(a) Boerhaave de Morb. Nerv. p. 820.

corripiantur." (*a*) Dr. Mead, in his learned treatiſe, *de imperio ſolis et lunæ*, furniſhes us with a very remarkable hiſtory of the epilepſy, cured by a diſcharge from the head, in conſequence of the application of a bliſter. A child about five years old, of a luſty and full habit of body, had convulſions ſo ſtrong and frequent, that her life was with difficulty ſaved by evacuants, and other medicines. She continued well for a few days, but was at the full of the moon, again attacked with a moſt violent fit; after which the diſeaſe regularly kept the ſame period with the tides. She continued in this ſtate fourteen days, that is, till the next great change of the moon, when a dry ſcab, the effect of an epiſpaſtic with which the whole *occiput* had been covered, broke out, and from the ſore iſſued a conſiderable quantity of limpid ſerum. This diſcharge was pro-

(*a*) Hippoc. de Morb. Sacro.

moted by proper applications; and the patient grew up to woman's eſtate, without ever ſuffering any return of the dreadful diſeaſe, under which ſhe had laboured. Celſus in the epilepſy recommends ſcarification, and the application of cupping glaſſes to the *occiput*; (a) and as this diſeaſe frequently ariſes, eſpecially in children, from plenitude, and a redundancy of humours in the head, a drain made from that part, may juſtly be regarded as a probable means of cure.

(a) Lib. 3. Cap. 23.

ESSAY

ESSAY V.

AN INQUIRY INTO THE RESEMBLANCE BETWEEN THE CHYLE AND MILK.

— *Probabilia conjectura ſequens.*

Cic. Tuſc. lib. 1.

ESSAY V.

AN INQUIRY INTO THE RESEMBLANCE BETWEEN CHYLE AND MILK.

THE properties of milk have with great ingenuity been inveſtigated, and with equal preciſion aſcertained, by ſeveral medical writers; and if the nature of the chyle were as well known, the ſubject of the preſent inquiry, would be obvious, and of eaſy ſolution. But as this fluid cannot, without great difficulty, be collected in ſufficient quantity, to undergo an experimental examination, it is almoſt impoſſible to determine its quali-ties,

ties, with any confiderable degree of certainty. Nor have I, in a great variety of authors which I have confulted, met with one experiment, which has been made immediately on the chyle, taken from the lacteal veffels. We muft therefore content ourfelves, with attempting to determine *à priori*, its nature and properties; that by comparing thefe with the known qualities of milk, fome probable conclufions at leaft may be deduced. And thefe conclufions may be confirmed by other arguments, drawn from facts and obfervations.

1. THE chyle muft neceffarily be compofed of the food we eat; which being mafticated in the mouth, and mixed with the fermentable faliva, is carried into the ftomach, where it receives the addition of the *fuccus gaftricus*, is further broke down, ferments, and paffes over the *pylorus* into the *duodenum*. Here it mixes with the bile, cyftic and hepatic, with the

the *ſuccus pancreaticus*, and the lymph which is thrown out, from the exhalant arteries, into the inteſtines. At length, if the animal feed chiefly upon vegetables, it is changed into a white and ſacharine fluid, which being imbibed by the lacteals, is carried into the courſe of circulation, to be further aſſimilated, animalized, and converted *in ſuccum et ſanguinem*.

The fluid thus formed, in all probability conſiſts of oil, mucilage, water, a coagulable part, and fixed air. That oil and mucilage enter into its compoſition, may be preſumed from the whiteneſs of its colour; for theſe two ſubſtances, when intimately combined with water, always put on that appearance. The exiſtence of a coagulable part in the chyle, is rather more uncertain; but I think there is ſome foundation for the hypotheſis. Our food is mixed in the *primæ viæ*, with a conſiderable quantity of lymph, which as it is composed of the serum of the blood, must be of a coagulable nature. And the mucilage contained in the aliment itself, possesses also in some degree the same property. So that we may with probability conclude, that the chyle is not destitute of a coagulable part. This coagulable part of the chyle, may possibly owe its origin, as much to the peculiar process of fermentation, which takes place in the *primæ viæ*, as to the animal fluids which are mixed with our food, in its passage through the stomach and small intestines. And this fermentation depends, in a great measure, on the nature of the aliments ingested. For it is observed, that a cow which feeds upon rank and watery grass, yields milk that contains very little *crassamentum*, and is therefore unfit for the purpose of making cheese. That fixed air enters into its composition, is acknowledged by every one, and has lately been very ingeniously illustrated,

illustrated, by the experiments of Dr. Macbride.

Boerhaave and other chemical writers, endeavour to explain the formation of chyle, by the instance of an emulsion, which is made by triturating any of the oleaginous vegetables with water. But the analogy between them is very imperfect, and perhaps only subsists in this single particular, that the white colour of each fluid arises from the mixture of oil and water, by the intervention of mucilage.

2. Milk consists of oil, mucilage, sugar, water, and air. The oil is obtained by a spontaneous separation, and is called cream. The mucilage is that coagulable part of which cheese is made. It has often been compared to the serum of the blood; but differs from it in this essential particular, that it is not coagulated by heat. The water contains a quantity of sugar,

ſugar, which may be ſeparated from it, by evaporating with a gentle heat, and cryſtallizing. That air is preſent in milk may be made evident to the ſenſes, by placing a quantity of it, previouſly heated, under the receiver of an air pump.

THE bare enumeration of the above particulars is ſufficient to ſhew, the ſimilitude which ſubſiſts between the two animal fluids, which form the ſubject of our preſent inquiry. And, if it could be ſatisfactorily aſcertained, that the properties, and component parts of the chyle are juſtly laid down, this exact reſemblance, would prove beyond all doubt, that they are one and the ſame. But, unfortunately, it cannot; and as my concluſion is founded upon hypotheſis alone, it is neceſſary to ſupport it by arguments, drawn from facts and obſervations.

1. MILK, as to its properties, depends upon the aliment. "*Pro vi et differentia*

tia aſſumptorum lac diverſum eſſe; ex illis enim chylus melior vel deterior, dulcis vel amarus, ex hoc tale lac; qualia enim ingeſta, talis chylus, qualis chylus, tale lac, aſſertum quotidiana confirmat experientia." (a) Dioſcorides relates, that the milk of goats which fed on the ſcammony plant and ſpurges, proved cathartic; and inſtances have been known, of an animal yielding bitter milk, from having eaten wormwood. (b) If a nurſe take a purgative, the infant will be purged; if ſhe drink wine or ſpirituous liquors, it will be intoxicated; (c) and I have been informed, from good authority, of one inſtance, where the eating of cabbage, or other flatulent vegetables, always gave the child the windy gripes. Milk, and the butter made from it, are found to differ greatly in colour, conſiſtence, taſte,

S and

(a) Crantz M. M. p. 80.

(b) *Vid.* Lewis's Mat. Med. p. 330.

(c) *Vid.* Boerhaav. Prælect. §. 690.

and ſmell, according to the food of the animal. Human milk is made yellow by taking ſaffron, bitter by wormwood, and impregnated with a garlic ſmell, by eating that root. (a) Boerhaave relates that thick ale, taken by a faſting nurſe, hath in a ſhort ſpace of time been diſcharged through the breaſts. (b) Theſe inſtances ſhew, that milk retains all the adventitious properties of the chyle; we may therefore conclude by analogy, that the natural and peculiar qualities of that fluid remain alſo unchanged.

2. The milk is proportioned in quantity, to the quantity of chyle. If the animal faſt for a long ſpace of time, neither chyle, nor milk is generated. The milk which is ſecreted immediately after taking in food, is found to be crude and indigeſted; becauſe it proceeds probably from the juices of the aliment, which are carried

(a) *Vid.* Neumann's Chemiſtry, p. 569. Notes.
(b) Prælect. §. 688.

ried into the ſyſtem by the abſorbent veſſels, before the chylous fermentation, if that expreſſion be allowable, is perfected. A nurſe yields the beſt milk about four hours after a meal; for by that time, the proceſs of digeſtion is fully compleated. In about eight hours, the chyle begins to be aſſimilated to the nature of the animal fluids, and then the milk aſſumes a yellowiſh colour, and acquires an offenſive taſte and ſmell. At length, when the chyle is converted into blood, the ſecretion from the breaſt, no longer bears any reſemblance to milk, but becomes acrid, fetid, and in every reſpect the reverſe of that mild, ſweet, and agreeable fluid.

3. THE ſacharine ſubſtance, which may be obtained from milk by inſpiſſation and cryſtallization, and the inflammable ſpirit, by fermentation and diſtillation, together with its aceſcent quality, in which it differs from all the other animal fluids, ſhew that the vegetable nature

of the chyle is unaltered in the veſſels of the breaſt. (a)

4. THAT the chyle may paſs through the courſe of circulation, without immediately mixing with the animal fluids, appears from the example of water, which is ſometimes ſecreted by the kidneys of hyſterical perſons, perfectly pure and inſipid. And that it realy does, is evident from venæſection: for the chyle hath been ſeen floating on blood, recently drawn from the arm. In the laſt ſtage of a diabetes, the urine manifeſtly points out the preſence of chyle in it, by its white colour, ſacharine taſte, and aceſcency. If it be kept in a cloſe veſſel ſeven or eight days, it will become ſour, and ferment ſtrongly with any of the mild alkaline ſalts. The learned Baron Van Swieten ſays, that a milky diſcharge hath

(a) IF an animal feed upon vegetable diet, the milk will be ſacharine and aceſcent; if upon animal, no ſugar will appear in that fluid, but on the contrary it will be putreſcent.

Vid. Young Diſſert. Inaug. Cap. viii. p. 55.

hath been obſerved in diarrhœas. *(a)* And Mr. Patch, in the Edinburgh Medical Eſſays, relates the caſe of a boy, from whoſe groin iſſued, through a ſmall and almoſt imperceptible orifice, four or five pints of a liquor like milk. *(b)*

5. THE remarkable laxity of the veſſels of the breaſts, aided by the power of ſuction, in diminiſhing the reſiſtance which the fluids might meet with in their paſſage through them, renders it probable, that the chyle may eaſily paſs into the breaſts, and be ſecreted there unchanged.

6. BUT the following hiſtory, which fell under the inſpection of a very celebrated phyſician, and was communicated to me by his friend and correſpondent, puts the matter almoſt beyond diſpute. I ſhall therefore conclude this inquiry with the detail of it. A girl about eight

(a) Van Swieten Comment. §. 1329.
(b) Edin. Med. Eſſays, Vol. 5.

eight years old, was tapped for an *aſcites.* She had alſo an univerſal *anaſarca*; and even her face was very much bloated, and exceedingly pale. Four quarts of liquor were drawn off, which was of a milky colour, full as white as milk mixed with an equal quantity of water. It would not coagulate by heat; but after ſtanding a day or two, it was covered with a kind of thin cream, and in a few days more, it ſmelt, and taſted ſour. The girl was greatly relieved by this evacuation; but the tumour of her belly, ſoon increaſed again to ſuch a degree, that it was neceſſary to renew the operation. A liquor the ſame as before, only ſomewhat more dilute, was drawn off, the ſwelling of her whole body ſubſided, and ſhe recovered her appetite and ſtrength. This girl before ſhe was attacked with theſe complaints, was very lively and active, and had a great appetite, in which ſhe was too much indulged. Probably by uſing violent exerciſe after a full meal, ſhe had ruptured ſome of the lacteals.

AN

APPENDIX.

Sapientis medici est, eorum locorum aquas ubi medicinam facit, convenienti examine probè scrutari, quo postea cum fructu, tam præservandi quam sanandi gratia, iis uti posset.

HOFFMAN.

EXPERIMENTS

AND

OBSERVATIONS

ON

WATER:

PARTICULARLY ON THE

HARD PUMP WATER

OF

MANCHESTER.

THE SECOND EDITION, REVISED AND ENLARGED.

—— *Sanctos ausus recludere fontes.*

VIRGIL.

THE

INTRODUCTION.

THE extensive influence of WATER on the health of mankind will, it is hoped, appear sufficiently evident from the following Essay. The author proposed to have enlarged the subject of it, by enquiring into the effects of hard and soft water on a variety of the common arts of life, such as Brewing, Malting, Dying, Bleaching, Tanning, &c. &c. But he found the subject too copious, to be reduced within the bounds which he had prescribed to himself; and that the prosecution of it, would too much abstract his attention from those favourite studies, which more immediately belong to his profession.

AN analysis of the waters, which are the objects of this enquiry, by means of evaporation, crystallization, &c. might perhaps

perhaps have aſcertained their contents with more minute exactneſs. But even this method is attended with ſome diſadvantages; becauſe heat decompoſes many ſaline bodies; and to determine the compoſition of the *reſiduum*, recourſe muſt have been had to the ſame chemical teſts, which the author employed in his experiments. And it would have been an almoſt endleſs trouble, thus to analyſe thirty different pump waters.

THIS Eſſay was intended only to be communicated to the ROYAL SOCIETY: And many of the experiments contained in it, have been read before that learned body. But the importance of the ſubject, and a deſire of rendering his little work more extenſively uſeful, hath induced the author to publiſh it. And he flatters himſelf, that he ſhall at leaſt be juſtified by the motives, if not by the ſucceſs of his undertaking.

MANCHESTER, Nov. 1, 1771.

EXPERIMENTS

AND

OBSERVATIONS

ON

WATER.

SECTION I.

IT is a maxim of the divine Hippocrates, that whoever would apply with ſucceſs to the ſtudy of phyſick, ſhould acquaint himſelf with every circumſtance relating to the ſituation of the place wherein he practiſes, the nature of the ſeaſons, the influence of the winds, and the particular qualities of the water. The laſt object is by far the moſt important; becauſe as a fixed and permanent

nent cauſe, its effects will be regular, uniform, and conſtant. For whether the ſimple element itſelf be uſed, or it be mixed with vinous liquors, or brewed into beer, it will ſtill retain in ſome meaſure its peculiar properties, and if impure, will gradually produce ſome morbid changes in the body. On the robuſt indeed, its action may perhaps be ſlow, and imperceptible; but the tender and valetudinary will find themſelves ſooner and more ſenſibly affected by it. Many of the diſeaſes of children, it is more than probable, owe their riſe to this neceſſary diluent and vehicle of their food. And if we conſider that numberleſs chronic diſorders have their foundation laid in the ſtate of infancy and childhood, the influence of water on the health of mankind will appear to be very extenſive, and deſerving of our ſtricteſt attention and regard. It would be no difficult matter to prove, that a conſiderable number of thoſe diſtempers, which from their being peculiar to certain people and places,

places, are termed endemic, are chiefly the effects of this powerful and active cause. Thus the inhabitants of the Alps, the Pyrenees, and of many other mountainous countries, are subject to a monstrous external swelling of the glands of the neck, owing as it is universally acknowledged, to the peculiar properties of the water they drink. (a) "As you advance towards Mount Cenis, says Mr. Sharp, in his excellent Letters from Italy, you find very few exempt from these tumours, which are so enormous, and of so loathsome an appearance, especially in ugly, ragged, half-starved old women, that the very sight of them turns the stomach. I was curious in my examination, whether any children are born with this malady upon them: I was informed, that there is no such instance; and even that the swelling never begins to form till towards two years of age; some examples of

(a) *Quis tumidum guttur miratur in Alpibus?*

Juvenal. Sat. 13.

of which I myself saw." (a) Nor is this distemper peculiar to the natives of those countries; for strangers become affected with it, after residing there a few years. (b) And such is the influence of custom on the common people, that they regard this blemish as a beauty, and even ridicule those who are destitute of it. At Rheims, the capital of the province of Champagne in France, there is hardly an aged person free from the *bronchocele*, owing to the drinking, till of late, the common water of their wells, which runs through a kind of chalky quarry, with which it is strongly charged. The same effect has been observed to arise from the abuse of sea water. (c) The inhabitants of the village of Steinseffein, in the district of Schmiderberg, are said to have freed themselves from this malady, by abstaining from certain fountains, which were

(a) Sharp's Letters, p. 298.

(b) Hoffman. Op. Tom. 6. p. 202.

(c) *Vid.* Lucas on Waters, Vol. 1, p. 29.

were obſerved to produce it. (a) In two cities of Hercynia, Wildeman, and Andreaſberg, which are built upon a large bed of minerals, ſcarcely a woman is to be found, who does not labour under ſtrumous ſwellings of the throat, occaſioned it is juſtly ſuppoſed, by the conſtant uſe of hard, metallic, and calcareous water. (b) The men too, in all probability, are not exempt from them; but as the female part of our ſpecies have more delicate conſtitutions, and eſpecially a much greater degree of laxity in their glandular ſyſtems than we have, the ſame cauſes which but ſlightly affect the one ſex, may prove highly injurious to the other. The people of Siberia, who live near the river Kirenga, which is remarkable for its impurity, are almoſt univerſally affected with ſcrophulous diſorders; and ſtrumous ſwellings are common, even amongſt the cattle of that country.

(a) Hoffman. Op. Tom. 6. p. 203.
(b) Id.

try. *(a)* It is worthy of obſervation, that horſes, by an inſtinctive ſagacity, always prefer ſoft water, to that which is hard. And when by neceſſity or inattention, they are confined to the latter, their coats become rough, and they are ſubject to the gripes.

HIPPOCRATES aſſerts that hard waters, which are unfit for boiling, dry and aſtringe the belly; and that ſuch as are ſtagnant and ill-ſcented, injure both the belly and ſpleen. *(b)* In confirmation of this, it may be obſerved, that in Minorca, where the water which the ſprings and rivulets afford, is often brackiſh, and always hard, obſtructions, indurations, and ſwellings of the abdominal viſcera, together with flatulency and indigeſtion, are the moſt common diſeaſes to which the inhabitants are ſubject. And it is remarkable, that large ſpleens and tumefied

(a) Comment. Lips. Tom. 2. p. 103.
(b) Hippoc. *de Aere, Aquis et Locis.*

mesied livers are not peculiar there to the human ſpecies, but are incident alſo to brutes; eſpecially to the ſheep, which feed on the eaſtern ſide of the iſland, where the waters are particularly brackiſh. *(a)* This ſhews the wiſdom of the ancients in examining the livers of the cattle which they offered in ſacrifice, wherever they propoſed to build a town, or to pitch a camp. If they proved to be firm and ſound, there they planned ſettlements, and erected fortifications. But on the contrary, if the livers appeared to be lax in their texture, or in any reſpect diſeaſed, they ſpeedily decamped; juſtly concluding, that the ſame food and water would produce a ſimilar effect, in human bodies. *(b)*

PLINY mentions a fountain in Æthiopia, about which a large quantity of native cinnabar was found, and which pro-

 duced

(a) Vid. Cleghorn on the Diſ. of Minorca.

(b) Vitruvius, Lib. 1. Cap. 4.

duced its deleterious effects chiefly on the brain. (a) And Athenæus speaks of a spring in Paphlagonia, to which the inhabitants of the country frequently resorted, which had an inebriating quality. Ovid poetically describes such waters in the following lines.

Cui non audita est obscenæ Salmacis undæ,
Æthiopesque lacus? quos si quis faucibus hausit,
Aut furit, aut patitur mirum gravitate soporem.

Metamorph. lib. 15, 317, 321.

THE *Plica Polonica*, a singular disease to which the inhabitants of Poland and Lithuania are subject, and which consists in a præternatural enlargement and convolution of the hair, is in part ascribed by a very celebrated writer, to the use of impure water. *Morbi hujus causa valde perplexa & difficilis videtur, nihilominus eam, quantum fieri poterit, indagare allabora-*

(a) Plin. Hist. lib. 31. c. 2.

allaborabimus. Primo multum ſordidum vitæ genus confert, cui hi populi addicti ſunt; dum raro crines pectunt in humidis et depreſſis locis dormiunt, et ſpiritum vini liberaliſſimè ingurgitant. Suum quoque ſymbolum AQUÆ *contribuunt; hinc non malè Gehema in Epiſtola ad Bontekoe, de Plica Polonica pag.* 10. *ſentit, hærere vitium in nonnullis Poloniæ aquis,* &c.

——— *Nos ſupponimus quoddam vitium hæreditarium, quod in nimia pororum et bulborum capillorum ſub cute in capite conſiſtit; unde ſuccus nutritius, craſſus, et glutinoſus, prava diæta ex* CRUDIS AQUIS *productus, calore, quem potus ſpiritus vini conciliat, urgetur ad tubulos capillorum, ex quorum poris exſudat, et monſtroſam illam intricationem efficit.* (*a*)—This ſuppoſition of the learned Hoffman is confirmed by the following aphoriſm of Sanctorius. Heavy water and a foggy air, convert the matter of perſpiration into an ichor,

 which

(*a*) *Vid.* Hoffman. Op. Tom. 6. p. 205.

which when retained in the body, induces a cachexy. *(a)*

Dr. Mead in the firſt edition of his Eſſay on Poiſons, relates the caſe of a lady, whoſe life was formerly imbittered by the frequent returns of violent colic pains, till ſhe was happily adviſed by her phyſician, not to drink, as ſhe uſually did, beer brewed with well water. And ſo evidently was the eſtabliſhment of her health owing to this caution, that the neglect of it was always attended with a return of her diſorder. A fact ſimilar to this is recorded by Van Helmont, of the monks belonging to a certain monaſtery near Bruſſels, who were always affected with the gripes by the water which they uſed, unleſs they corrected its effects by boiling wild carrot ſeeds in their beer. *(b)*

The

(a) Sanctor. Med. Stat. Sect. 2. Aph. 6.

(b) Helmont's Lithiaſis.—*Vid.* alſo Hale's Stat. Eſſays, Vol. 2. p. 248.

THE *Elephantiaſis* is endemial amongſt the Egyptians, *(a)* and is aſcribed by Galen and Avicena to the uſe of the impure waters of the Nile. Lucretius alſo adopted the ſame opinion, as appears by the following lines.

Eſt Elephas Morbus, qui propter flumina Nili
Gignitur Ægypto in medio. ——

IT is an opinion which the father of phyſick firſt advanced, and which has been almoſt univerſally adopted by his followers, and hath remained till lately uncontroverted, that the ſtone and gravel are generated by the uſe of hard water. *Damnantur imprimis fontes*, ſays Pliny, *quorum Aquæ decoctæ, craſſis obducunt vaſa cruſtis.* *(b)* And from this quality, which the waters of certain ſprings poſſeſs, of depoſiting a large earthy ſediment,

(a) Alpinus de Med. Ægypt. Lib. 1. Cap. 4
(b) Lib. 31. c. 3.

ment, either in the aquæducts through which they are conveyed, or in the veſſels in which they are boiled or preſerved, it was obvious to infer, that in paſſing through the kidneys, and eſpecially whilſt retained in the bladder, they would let fall their groſſer particles, which by the continued appoſition of freſh matter, connected by the animal gluten, and compacted by the muſcular action of that organ, would in time form a *Calculus*, ſufficiently large to produce a train of the moſt excruciating ſymptoms. And this reaſoning *à priori*, has been ſuppoſed to be confirmed by facts and experience; for not to mention the authority of Hippocrates, Dr. Liſter has obſerved, that the inhabitants of Paris, are peculiarly ſubject to the ſtone in the bladder. *(a)* And

(a) Vid. Liſter's Journey to Paris.

NICHOLAS DE BLEGNY has related the hiſtory of one who was diſſected at Paris, in whom the Pylorus, a great part of the Duodenum, and the ſtomach itſelf, were found incruſtated with a ſtony matter, to the thickneſs of a finger's

And it is well known, that the water of the river Seine, with which that city is ſupplied, is ſo impregnated with calcareous matter, as to incruſtate, and in a ſhort time to choak up the pipes through which it runs. But on the other hand it is objected, that the human *Calculus* is of animal origin, and by chemical analyſis, appears to bear very little analogy to the ſtony concretions of water. And though it is allowed, that more perſons are cut for the ſtone in the hoſpitals at Paris, than in moſt other places, yet upon enquiry it is found, that many of thoſe patients come from different provinces, and from towns and villages far diſtant from the Seine.

I WILL not preſume to decide this diſputed point: but if I may be allowed to indulge a conjecture, I ſhould ſuppoſe, that though this diſeaſe may chiefly depend

finger's breadth. Zodiac. Med. Gallic. A. D. 1679. Mens. Feb. Obſ. 3.

pend upon a peculiar diſpoſition to concrete in the animal fluids, which in many inſtances is hereditary, and in no inſtance can with certainty be imputed to any particular cauſe; yet, hard water is at leaſt negatively favourable to this *diatheſis*, by having no tendency to diminiſh it. The urine of the moſt healthy perſon, is generally loaded with terreous matter, capable, in favourable circumſtances, of forming a *Calculus*; as is evident from the thick cruſt which it depoſits, on the ſides of the veſſels in which it is contained. And it ſeems as if nature intended by this excretion, to diſcharge all the ſuperfluous ſalts of the blood, together with thoſe earthy particles, which are either derived from our aliment, and fine enough to paſs through the lacteals, though inſuperable by the powers of circulation, or which ariſe from the abraſion of the ſolids, or from the diſſolution of the red globular part of our fluids. Now water, whether uſed as nature preſents us with it, or mixed ed with wine, or taken under the form of beer or ale, is the great diluter, vehicle, and *menſtruum* both of our food, and of the ſaline, earthy, and recrementitious parts of the animal juices. And it is more or leſs adapted to the performance of theſe offices, in proportion to its degree of purity. For it muſt appear evident to the moſt ordinary underſtanding, that a *menſtruum* already loaded, and perhaps ſaturated, with different contents, cannot act ſo powerfully as one which is free from all ſenſible impregnation. Nor is this reaſoning founded upon theory alone; *(a)* for it is obſerved, that MALVERN

(a) A gentleman of this place, who had been long ſubject to nephritic complaints, and often voided ſmall ſtones, was adviſed to refrain from his own-pump water, which is uncommonly hard, and to drink conſtantly the ſofter water of a neighbouring ſpring. And this change alone, without the uſe of any medicine, hath rendered the returns of his diſorder much leſs frequent and painful. A lady alſo, much affected with the gravel, was induced by the peruſal of the firſt edition of this eſſay, to try the effect of ſoft water; and by the conſtant uſe of it, ſhe has remained two years entirely free from her diſorder.

VERN WATER, which iſſues from a ſpring in Worceſterſhire, remarkable for its uncommon purity, hath the property of diſſolving the little ſabulous ſtones, which are often voided in nephritic complaints. And the ſolution too, which is a proof of its being complete, is perfectly colourleſs. Hence this water is drunk with great advantage in diſorders of the urinary paſſages. And during the uſe of it, the patient's urine is generally limpid, and ſeldom depoſits any ſandy ſediment. Yet notwithſtanding this appearance of tranſparency, it is certainly at ſuch times, loaded with impurities, which are ſo diluted and diſſolved as not to be viſible. For it is attended with a ſtrong and fœtid ſmell, exactly reſembling that of aſparagus. *(a)* Hoffman mentions a pure, light, ſimple

(a) Vid. Dr. Wall on Malvern Water.

IN Nephritic caſes, diſtilled water would be an excellent ſubſtitute for Malvern Water, as the following experiment evinces.

Two

ſimple water in the principality of Henneberg, in Germany, which is remarkable for its efficacy in the ſtone and gravel; and a water of ſimilar virtues, was diſcovered not many years ago, in the black foreſt, near Oſterod, which upon examination did not afford a ſingle grain of mineral matter. Indeed it is worthy of obſervation, that moſt of the ſprings, which were formerly held in great eſteem, and were called *holy wells*, are very pure, and yield little or no ſediment.

THESE obſervations are ſufficient to ſhew the utility and importance of the following chemical enquiry, into the nature and properties of the PUMP WATER of

Two fragments of the ſame Calculus, nearly of equal weights, were immerſed, the one in three ounces of diſtilled water, the other in three ounces of hard pump water. The phials were hung up cloſe together, in a kitchen chimney, at a convenient diſtance from the fire. After fourteen days maceration, the calculi were taken out, and carefully dried by a very gentle heat. The former, viz. that which had been immerſed in diſtilled water, was diminiſhed in its weight a grain and half; the latter had loſt only half a grain.

of MANCHESTER. I ſhall therefore proceed to lay before the reader the moſt intereſting of my experiments on this ſubject, with ſuch inferences as are obviouſly deducible from them.

EXPERIMENT I.

NEAR thirty different pump waters, moſt of them collected from pumps common to a whole neighbourhood, were chemically examined. They all curdled ſoap; the volatile alkali occaſioned a precipitation in many of them; the fixed alkali in all of them; and they became quite milky with a ſolution of *ſacharum ſaturni*. The infuſion of galls produced no change in their colour; but ſyrup of violets turned moſt of them green.

EXPERIMENT II.

A THREE ounce phial, after being carefully counterpoiſed in a very nice balance, was filled to the brim with diſtilled

tilled pump water, which weighed twenty one drachms and fifty grains. The ſame phial, exactly balanced as before, was then filled to the brim with my own pump water, of the ſame temperature with the diſtilled water, which weighed twenty one drachms and fifty ſix grains. (a) Several other pump waters were examined in the ſame way, and very little difference was found in their ſpecific gravities. The water of a pump belonging to a public brewery in this place, weighed indeed, in the quantity above-mentioned, only twenty one drachms and fifty three grains. But on enquiry I learned, that this water is contained in a reſervoir, ſupplied by means of pipes, either from the rain which falls in the neighbouring grounds, or from the ſuperficial ſprings which run through them.

FROM

(a) THIS experiment was afterwards tried by the hydroſtatical balance, with no other difference in the reſult, but a ſmall fraction of a grain.

From the foregoing experiments it is obvious, that the pump water of Manchester is in general very impure. It is impregnated with a large quantity of selenite; an earthy, astringent salt, composed of the vitriolic, nitrous, or marine acid, and calcareous earth; and at the same time contains no inconsiderable proportion of alum, as may be reasonably inferred, from the green colour which it strikes with syrup of violets. For though it be acknowledged, that Buxton, Bristol, Pyrmont, Spa, and other springs, which are not aluminous, produce a similar effect, yet these are all impregnated with mineral alkali, or with other substances, of which the Manchester pump water appears to be destitute, by the chemical tests employed in its examination. *(a)* But what puts this conclusion beyond

(a) Dr. Lewis asserts in his *Materia Medica*, p. 71. "that the blue juices of vegetables are changed red by alum;" and again in his excellent notes on Neumann's Chemistry,

beyond diſpute is, that the earth of alum is frequently found in the wells of this town. I have now in my poſſeſſion ſome of this earth, which by the addition of oil of vitriol, has been converted into true alum —From the ſecond experiment it is evident, that a quart of water contains upwards of ſixty grains of adventitious matter; and ſuppoſing this quantity to be daily conſumed, in one way or other, by every individual, which is a moderate

U compu-

Chemiſtry, p. 252. " that ſyrup of violets is changed red by waters impregnated with alum." The fact was otherwiſe in my trials; for two grains of alum diſſolved in an ounce of diſtilled water, ſtruck a pea green with twenty drops of the ſame ſyrup of violets, which was uſed in the above recited experiments. A tea-ſpoonful of lime water added to a part of the ſolution, conſiderably deepened the green colour; whereas two drops of elixir of vitriol produced in the other part a ſenſible, though faint redneſs. A ſolution of alum alſo in lime water was turned at once into a deep green, by the addition of a ſmall portion of ſyrup of violets. The lime water was added in the firſt experiment, to render the water employed more analogous to the hard, calcareous pump water of Mancheſter.

IN a later trial I have found that the blue or purple juice of radiſhes is changed to a red, ſo ſlight however as barely

computation, about forty ſix ounces troy weight, of crude, earthy, indigeſtible, and by no means inactive ſalts, will in the courſe of twelve months, be received into the body. And how pernicious this may be to health, thoſe can beſt conceive, who know the powerful influence of ſlight, but continued cauſes on the human frame. (a) It would be foreign to

barely to be perceptible, by a ſolution of alum in water. But this does not invalidate my concluſion, that many of the pump waters of Mancheſter are aluminous, becauſe they are turned green by an admixture of ſyrup of violets. For it appears, that a ſolution of alum produced a green colour in the ſame ſyrup of violets, which was employed in the before-mentioned experiment. And to ſecure againſt all fallacy, I repeated that experiment ſeveral times: nor had I reaſon to ſuſpect the genuineneſs of the ſyrup, as it was prepared at the Apothecary's Hall, and never failed to become red, on the addition of an acid. The reſult of it is alſo corroborated by the teſtimony of Neumann, who aſſerts, that the common ſorts of alum change the ſyrup of violets green. Dr. Rutty ſays, that ſyrup of violets when new is turned red, but when kept ſome time green, by alum.

(a) *Quid magis eſt ſaxo durum? Quid mollius unda?*
Dura tamen molli ſaxa cavantur aqua.

Ovid.

to my preſent purpoſe, to enter into a detail of the endemic diſeaſes of Mancheſter. But one obſervation I cannot omit, that the inhabitants of this place are peculiarly ſubject to glandular obſtructions, and ſcrophulous ſwellings. And that water loaded with aſtringent, earthy ſalts, hath a direct tendency to produce ſuch complaints, has been already I hope fully evinced.

BUT hard and impure water may be conſidered in a further view as injurious to the human body. It was before obſerved, that this univerſal *menſtruum* is deſigned by nature to be the diluter, vehicle, and ſolvent both of our food, and of the recrementitious parts of the animal fluids. And in the performance of theſe ſalutary offices, it immediately promotes the general health of the body, and at the ſame time counteracts the influence of various cauſes of diſeaſe. The Spaniards, it is ſaid, are for the moſt part exempt from the itch and the ſcurvy, notwith-

 ſtanding

ſtanding they indulge themſelves in the daily uſe of pork, the leaſt perſpirable of all foods. And the reaſon aſſigned for this remarkable fact is, that the air of Spain is clear, thin, and ſerene, and the water light, pure, and wholeſome. *(a)* Hence the minuteſt ſeries of veſſels are continued permeable and unobſtructed, perſpiration is free and copious, all the excretions are duly and regularly performed, and every thing putrid and acrimonious is carried out of the ſyſtem, before it has time to create diſturbance or diſorder. But water impregnated with auſtere, earthy, and indigeſtible ſalts, is ill qualified to anſwer theſe important ends. Already nearly ſaturated with its heterogeneous contents, it is rendered leſs capable

(a) Vid. Hoffmani Opera, Tom 6. p. 204.

HERODOTUS, whoſe teſtimony is not always to be depended upon, relates that in Æthiopia the inhabitants live to be an hundred and twenty years old, that they eat fleſh, and drink milk; that the water of the country is ſo light, that nothing will float upon it, not even wood, and that the uſe of this water makes them long lived.

Lib. 3. c. 125.

capable of diſſolving our food, of mingling uniformly with our fluids, or penetrating the fineſt ramifications of the vaſcular ſyſtem, and of paſſing off copiouſly and eaſily by the ſeveral emunctories. And thus it becomes negatively the cauſe of diſeaſes.

IT is therefore of the utmoſt conſequence, where nature hath denied the benefit of pure water, to diſcover ſome means of correcting its pernicious qualities. And with this view the following experiments were made.

EXPERIMENT III.

A STRONG ſolution of ſalt of tartar was inſtilled into hard pump water, till no lacteſcency enſued. The ſame experiment was repeated with a ſmaller quantity of *ſal tartari*, ſo as not to deſtroy the inſipidity of the water; but the ſoftening effect of the vegetable alkali, was then ſcarcely perceptible. Hence it appears that the Manchester pump waters, are too hard to be much improved in this way, without rendering them offensive to the palate.

EXPERIMENT IV.

To half an ounce of hard pump water, just boiled, were added five drops of a solution of *sacharum saturni*. To an equal quantity of the same water unboiled, were also added five drops. The boiled became much less milky than the cold water. But supposing this effect to arise from the heat of the water, I poured half an ounce of it into a glass, and when cold, instilled five drops of the solution of sugar of lead into it as before, without any increase of its lactescency. I then took equal quantities, viz. half an ounce of unboiled water, and of water which had been boiled over a brisk fire during the space of twenty minutes, and poured into each a few drops of the solution of *sacharum saturni*. The raw water became twice as milky

milky as the boiled water, and depoſited a much larger ſediment. And I thought the water which had been boiled twenty minutes, was leſs changed by the addition of ſugar of lead, than that which had undergone only a ſlight coction. Ten drops of *ſp. ſal. ammon. vol.* added to half an ounce of raw ſpring water, turned it milky; but when added to an equal quantity of the ſame water which had been boiled twenty minutes, no change was produced. Three grains of fixed alkali *(ſal tartari)* diſſolved in half an ounce of the ſame boiled water, occaſioned no ſenſible cloudineſs; but when mixed with an equal quantity of raw water, a great lacteſcency and copious precipitation immediately enſued. The boiled water ſtill continued to break and curdle with ſoap, though in a leſs degree than the ſame water unboiled. The former alſo felt to the touch much ſofter than the latter.

THIS experiment clearly demonſtrates,

 that

that hard water is freed from ſome of its earthy ſalts, and rendered conſiderably ſofter by boiling. And it appears likewiſe, that the coction ſhould be continued ſome time, in order to produce its full effect. Dr. Heberden is indeed of a contrary opinion; for notwithſtanding he acknowledges, that the unneutralized lime-ſtone and ſelenite is ſeparated by boiling from pump water, yet he thinks it becomes more ſtrongly impregnated with the ſaline matter, and conſequently leſs ſalutary. But in this inſtance, the Doctor appears not to reaſon with his uſual judgment and accuracy; and I apprehend, his obſervation is neither confirmed by analogy, nor ſupported by experiment. For though heat generally increaſes the diſſolving power of any *menſtruum*, at the ſame time it tends, in many inſtances, to deſtroy the texture, and diſunite the component parts of the ſolvend. Thus hot water ſuſpends a much larger quantity of nitre than cold water; but if the ſolution be boiled over the

the fire, a conſiderable portion of the ſalt-petre will be diſſipated. If then the nitrous acid be volatiliſed and ſeparated from its alkali by coction, may we not juſtly infer, that it will be diſengaged by the ſame cauſe from an earthy baſis, to which it bears comparatively but a weak affinity? And the ſame reaſoning may be applied with equal force to the volatile vitriolic or muriatic acids, which in all probability fly off by means of the boiling heat, leaving behind them an indiſſoluble, petrifying earth, that ſubſides to the bottom, and incruſts the veſſel.

EXPERIMENT V.

A quantity of hard pump water, which had paſſed through a filtering ſtone, when compared with the ſame water unfiltered, was found to be conſiderably ſoftened. Each curdled with ſoap, but the former in a leſs degree than the latter. The volatile alkali occaſioned no cloudineſs in the filtered water, but a viſible one in the

the other: The fixed alkali produced a precipitation in both, leſs however in the former, than in the latter; and the ſolution of *ſacharum ſaturni* rendered the unfiltered water much more lacteſcent, than that which had ſoaked through the filtering ſtone.

These two experiments point out an eaſy and obvious method of purifying hard water, by freeing it in ſome meaſure, from the unneutraliſed ſelenite, and groſſer ſalts which it contains. The water ſhould firſt be boiled for the ſpace of fifteen or twenty minutes, then paſſed through the filtering ſtone, and afterwards ſuffered to ſtand a few hours, till it has attracted from the atmoſphere a due proportion of air. Thus it will be rendered tolerably pure, ſalutary, and potable, and at the ſame time much better adapted to a variety of culinary uſes. If a filtering ſtone cannot eaſily be provided, the following ſimple contrivance may be ſubſtituted in its room. Let a large funnel be be made of wood, fill the narrow neck of it with ſponge; above the ſponge ſpread a layer of ſand and gravel; cover this with a piece of thick flannel, and place over the whole another layer of ſand, leaving ſufficient room for the water, which is to be filtered. Care muſt be taken to change the ſponge, ſand, &c. as often as they become loaded with the impurities of the water. *(a)*

EXPERIMENT VI.

MR. BOYLE aſſerts that ſome pump waters, barely by ſtanding a few days, will become ſoft enough to mix uniformly with ſoap. *(b)* A quantity of hard pump water was therefore expoſed to the ſun and air, but ſo as to be ſheltered from the rain, for the ſpace of a week. It curdled with ſoap, and became as milky with a few drops of ſugar of lead, as water

(a) Vid. Lind on the health of ſeamen, p. 92.

(b) Boyle's Works, Shaw's Edit. Vol. 1. p. 141.

ter juſt drawn from the well. The volatile alkali indeed, produced no cloudineſs in it, and this was the only mark which it afforded of being in the leaſt degree ſoftened.

EXPERIMENT VII.

A STRONG infuſion of malt was not more miſcible with ſoap, than the boiled water with which it was prepared; nor did it ſuffer a leſs precipitation on the addition of a few grains of *ſacharum ſaturni*.

EXPERIMENT VIII.

STRONG table beer, drawn from the barrel about ten days after it had been brewed, curdled with ſoap as much as the hard water boiled, which was employed in its preparation.

HENCE it appears that fermentation hath not the power of ſoftening hard water;

ter; and that the wholeſomeneſs of malt liquors, muſt greatly depend upon the purity of the water which is uſed in brewing them. This coincides with the following obſervation of Hoffman: *Bonitas cereviſiarum primò à ſalubri aqua dependet. Quo ſalubrior aqua fontana eſt, eo præſtantiorem exhibet cereviſiam; & quo ſubtilior aqua, eo plus ingredientia extrahit, eoque melius fermenteſcit.* (a) As a ſeaſon for brewing, the month of March is preferable to October, becauſe the ſprings are then increaſed by the winter rains, and are proportionably ſofter and more ſalutary.

EXPERIMENT IX.

STRONG infuſions of green and bohea tea in boiled hard water, curdled with ſoap, and were as much changed by the addition of ſugar of lead, as the boiled water itſelf. So that theſe faſhionable and

(a) Hoffman. Op. Vol. 1. p. 113.

and favourite articles of diet, notwithſtanding the ſoft taſte which they communicate to the hardeſt water, do not really alter or improve its nature. It were well however, if tea could be conſiaered in this reſpect merely as innocent or uſeleſs; but it imparts many pernicious qaalities to its aqueous vehicle; and the daily uſe of it, by inſenſible degrees enfeebles the conſtitution, and brings on a train of nervous diſorders.

EXPERIMENT X.

Two or three pieces of common brick were ſteeped four days, in a baſon full of diſtilled water. The water was then decanted off, and examined by various chemical teſts. It was immiſcible with ſoap, ſtruck a lively green with ſyrup of violets, was rendered ſlightly lacteſcent by the volatile alkali, and quite milky by the fixed alkali, and by a ſolution of *ſacharum ſaturni*. The infuſion of tormentil root produced no change in it.

EXPERI-

EXPERIMENT XI.

AN experiment ſimilar to the former was tried with a rough piece of freeſtone, (*ſaxum arenarium*) which did not appear to have communicated any impregnation to a baſon full of diſtilled water, in which it had been ſeveral days immerſed.

THE 10th experiment affords a ſtriking proof of the impropriety of lining wells with brick, a practice very common in many places, and which cannot fail of rendering the water hard and unwholeſome. Clay generally contains a variety of heterogeneous matters. The coloured loams often participate of bitumen, and the ocher of iron: Sand and calcareous earth are ſtill more common ingredients in their compoſition; and the experiments of Mr. Geoffroy and Mr. Pott prove, that the earth of alum alſo, may in large quantity be extracted from them. Now as clay is expoſed to the open

open air for a long ſpace of time, is then moulded into bricks, and burnt, this proceſs reſembles in many reſpects that by which the alum-ſtone is prepared. And it is probable, that the white efflo-reſcence, which is frequently obſervable on the ſurface of new bricks, is of an aluminous nature. *(a)*

It hath long been a prevailing opinion, that water flowing through leaden pipes, acquires certain noxious qualities. Hippocrates, and his commentator Galen, expreſſly condemn the uſe of ſuch water; and Vitruvius in his treatiſe on Architecture, remonſtrates ſtrongly againſt that means of conveying water. *Multo ſalubrior ex tubulis aqua quam per fiſtulas: quod per plumbum videtur eſſe ideo vitioſa, quod ex eo ceruſſa*

(a) The long expoſure of clay to the air, before it is moulded into bricks, the ſulphureous exhalations of the pit coal uſed in burning it, together with the ſuffocating and bitumenous vapour which ariſes from the ignited clay itſelf, ſufficiently account for the combination of a vitriolic acid with the earth of alum.

cerussa nascitur: hæc autem dicitur nocens esse corporibus humanis. Itaque minimè fistulis plumbeis aqua duci videtur, si volumus eam habere salubrem. (a) Neumann, whose authority as a chemist is of great weight, gives it as his opinion, that the waters conveyed by pipes may corrode some of the matter of the pipe or of its cement, and thus contract disagreeable qualities. And he assures us, that having examined the aquæducts at Rome, those between Marly and Versailles in France, and those by which London is supplied with the New-river water, he found them in some places liable to this inconvenience. (b) Doctor Falconer in his ingenious and useful Treatise on the Bath waters, informs us that the leaden cistern, which serves as a reservoir for the spring at its first rise, is very much corroded on the inside, as appears by the long furrows

 which

(a) Vitruvius, lib. 8. c. 7.

(b) Neumann's Chem. by Lewis, p. 248.

which are viſible in every part of it. And he, with great propriety, imputes the failure of cure, of many bowel diſorders, and the obſtinate coſtiveneſs ſo much complained of on drinking the Bath waters, in ſome meaſure to this cauſe. *(a)* Baron Van Swieton alſo relates, " *Vidi integram familiam hoc morbo (ſcilicet Colica Pictonum) laboraſſe, dum ad culinares uſus adhibebatur aqua, in magno receptaculo plumbeo collecta, & diu hærens.*" But a celebrated writer, who has lately favoured the public with an excellent Treatiſe on the Poiſon of Lead, thinks the caution of Vitruvius and of Galen unneceſſary, except in ſuch caſes where a quantity of vegetable acid might be ſuppoſed to render the metal diſſoluble in water. *(b)* I cannot however agree with him in this opinion, notwithſtanding

(a) THE waters of the Hot Bath are obſerved rather to open, than bind the body. The reſervoir there is made of ſtone.

Falconer on Bath Waters, p. 184.

(b) Vid. Medical Tranſactions, No. 13.

ing his experiments at firſt ſight appear to be ſo concluſive. For I apprehend the water he employed in his trials, either contained no acid, or that the acid was combined with other ſubſtances, by which it was more powerfully attracted than by lead. This metal diſſolves very readily in weak *aqua fortis*, in the volatile vitriolic acid, or in oil of vitriol well diluted with water. (a) And from Dr. Cullen's table of Elective Attractions it appears, that the laſt of theſe acids has a much ſtronger affinity with lead, than with the earthy baſis of alum. As ſpring waters are therefote ſo frequently found to be aluminous, may we not with reaſon ſuſpect, that in their paſſage through leaden pipes, the vitriolic acid will depoſit the earth with which it was combined, and diſſolve ſome portion of the metal. And thus the fountain will become impregnated with a metallic ſalt, of the moſt

 poiſon-

(a) Shaw's Notes to Boerhaave's Chem. Vol. 1. p. 85.

poiſonous and deleterious quality. It is a common obſervation that hard water renders pewter black; and this in all probability ariſes from a ſolution of the lead and tin, of which this mixed metal is compoſed. But as a point of ſo much importance to the health of mankind, ought to reſt on better evidence than theoretical reaſoning, the following experiment was made in order to determine, whether water impregnated with alum be capable of diſſolving lead.

EXPERIMENT XII.

Two clean and bright bits of lead, weighing 327 grains were immerſed ſixteen days in a phial of water, in which a drachm of alum had been previouſly diſſolved. The volatile tincture of ſulphur produced no blackneſs in this water, until a few drops of the ſolution of *ſacharum ſaturni* were added to it, and then a duſky colour immediately ſucceeded. The bits

of

of lead carefully wiped and dried, were not found to have ſuffered any ſenſible loſs of weight.

THE ſame experiment was repeated with hard, aluminous pump water. I conceived, that the lead had communicated ſomewhat of a ſweetiſh taſte to the water; but when a few drops of the volatile tincture of ſulphur were inſtilled into it, it did not exhibit any appearance of a ſaturnine impregnation; nor had the bits of lead loſt any part of their weight.

THOUGH the reſult of this experiment ſeems to overturn the theory before advanced, yet it does not afford me full conviction, that lead is totally inſoluble in aluminous waters. For the volatile tincture of ſulphur may not perhaps, in every inſtance, be a certain criterion of the preſence of this poiſonous mineral, as I have proved, that green vitriol is not of the aſtringency of vegetables.(*a*) Beſides a proportion of lead, too inconſiderable to be detected by any chemical examination, may poſſibly, in irritable habits, and under certain delicate circumſtances, prove highly injurious to health. (*b*) This is confirmed by the account which Doctor Tronchin has given of the Colic of Amſterdam, the cauſe of which long eluded the reſearches of the learned: At laſt however it was diſcovered to ariſe from the uſe of water, ſlightly impregnated with lead. But conſcious of the influence of a preconceived hypotheſis, I have fairly ſtated both the reaſons and facts, relating to this point, and ſhall leave the deciſion concerning them to the more unbiaſſed judgment of the reader. The uſe of leaden pumps however may be pernicious, though the conveyance of water through pipes of this metal ſhould not

(*a*) Experiments on Aſtringents, 2 Edit. p. 150.

(*b*) *Vid.* Dr. Falconer on Bath Waters, p. 187.

not be esteemed so: For by the friction of the bucket against the sides of the pump, some portion of lead will be rubbed off, and suspended in the water. (a)

(a) THOUGH it be foreign to my present subject, I cannot omit this opportunity of cautioning against the practice of cleaning wine bottles with leaden shot. It frequently happens, I am persuaded, through inattention, that some of the little pellets are left behind; and when wine or beer is again poured into the bottles, this mineral poison will slowly dissolve, and impregnate those vinous liquors with its deleterious qualities. The sweetness which is sometimes perceived in Red Port Wine, may arise from this cause, when such an adulteration is neither designed nor suspected.

SECTION II.

FROM the ſubject of this experimental enquiry into the different properties of hard and ſoft water, we are naturally led to conſider their influence on many of the operations of PHARMACY. And we ſhall find, that the moſt innocent vehicle, is alſo the moſt powerful *menſtruum* for extracting the virtues of medicines.

EXPERIMENT XIII.

Two drachms of green tea, were ſeparately macerated without heat, an equal length of time, the one in three ounces of hard pump water, and the other in the ſame quantity of diſtilled water. The latter

latter infusion had a more bitter taste, and struck a much deeper black than the former, with three grains of *sal martis*..

EXPERIMENT XIV.

A DRACHM of bark finely powdered, was macerated two days, without heat, in three ounces of distilled water; and the same quantity, during the same space of time, in three ounces of hard pump water. The infusion made with distilled water, was of a paler colour than the other, but yet tasted more intensely bitter, although somewhat less rough and styptic. Two grains of *sal martis* were added to half an ounce of each infusion, carefully filtered. The latter struck a much deeper black than the former.

DISAPPOINTED in the result of this experiment, I repeated it again, but with nearly the same success as before. Twenty drops of a strong solution of *sal martis*, produced at first no sensible change in half

half an ounce of the infuſion made with diſtilled water, whilſt the ſame number of drops, almoſt inſtantly ſtruck an inky blackneſs with the other infuſion, prepared with hard pump water. By degrees indeed the former aſſumed a duſky hue, but after ſtanding many hours, did not half equal the blackneſs of the latter.

EXPERIMENT XV.

THIRTY drops of a ſolution of alum in lime water were inſtilled into half an ounce of the infuſion of bark, made with diſtilled water. By this addition the ſame quantity of *ſal martis* employed in the laſt experiment, immediately produced a very duſky colour; and in leſs than an hour, the mixture aſſumed an inky blackneſs.

EXPERIMENT XVI.

Two drachms of tormentil root bruiſed, were macerated in equal quantities, viz.

viz. three ounces of hard pump water, and of diſtilled water, during the ſpace of twenty four hours. The latter infuſion was of a deeper orange colour, than the former, and had a rougher and more ſtyptic taſte. But when twenty drops of a ſolution of *ſal martis* were added to equal portions of each infuſion, an inky blackneſs, to all appearance preciſely the ſame, enſued in both.

EXPERIMENT XVII.

An experiment ſimilar to the former was tried with Aleppo galls, by macerating two drachms of their powder in equal quantities of hard pump water, and of diſtilled water; but the reſult was ſomewhat different. I could not by comparing their taſtes, determine which infuſion was moſt aſtringent or ſtyptic. The one made with diſtilled water was of a paler colour than the other; yet it ſtruck a much deeper black with green vitriol.

EXPERI-

EXPERIMENT XVIII.

EQUAL quantities of Peruvian bark powdered, were macerated without heat forty eight hours, in three ounces of hard pump water, and of the ſame pump water boiled. The latter infuſion had a ſtronger taſte of the *cortex*, but did not ſtrike ſo deep a black with the ſolution of *ſal martis*.

FROM theſe experiments it may be inferred that ſoft water, and eſpecially diſtilled water, acts far more powerfully as a *menſtruum* on vegetable bitters and aſtringents, than hard pump water. And the concluſion may in all probability, be extended to many other claſſes of vegetables. The fourteenth experiment indeed, ſeems at firſt view to prove that the Peruvian bark yields its aſtringency more perfectly to hard, than to ſoft water; but the ſucceeding experiment ſhews the fallacy of this inference. For the addition of of thirty drops of a ſolution of alum in lime water, could not give any real increaſe to the ſtrength of an infuſion of the *cortex*, previouſly prepared; although it enabled it to ſtrike a deeper black with green vitriol. But from this curious fact we may conclude, that hard, aluminous waters are likely to anſwer beſt in the dying of black; and this is confirmed by the obſervation of Dr. Lewis, that alum heightens the colour of the watery tinctures of madder and brazil. (*a*) Mr. Chambers, in his uſeful Dictionary, informs us, that well-water is preferred for dying red, and other colours which require aſtringency, and alſo for dying ſtuffs of a looſe contexture, ſuch as callico, fuſtian, and cotton. Doctor Rutty alſo found by experiment, that hard water extracts a tincture of a deeper hue than ſoft water, from logwood, brazil, ſena, rhuburb, and cale.

IT

(*a*) *Vid.* Neumann's Chem. by Lewis, p. 187.

It is found that hard, calcareous waters render the mixture of resinous bodies, by the intervention of mucilage of gum arabic, difficult and sometimes impracticable. (a) This naturally led me to conceive, that soft or distilled water, might possibly dissolve those substances without the assistance of any medium, or at least with a much smaller proportion of gum, than is commonly employed. On suggesting this hint to a sensible and ingenious Apothecary of this place, he very obligingly undertook to make the experiments for me, and has sent me the following account of the result of them, which I shall deliver in his own words. The letter contains some further trials, which do not relate to the present subject; but as they lead to several useful and important conclusions, I shall without any apology insert them.

June

(a) *Vid.* Lond. Med. Observ. Vol. 1. p. 435.

June 29, 1768.

DEAR SIR,

I Have made the experiments you desired of dissolving resinous substances in distilled and common pump water, the result of which seems to be much in favour of the former.

ONE scruple of balsam of tolu, rubbed with half an ounce of distilled rain water, added gradually to it, for fifteen minutes, formed a mixture, which on standing about a minute subsided, but reunited by shaking: Being set by a few days, the balsam became a concrete mass, not again miscible by shaking up the bottle.

THE same quantity required more trituration to mix it with common pump water. The mixture was not kept.

ONE scruple of the same, rubbed with fifteen grains of gum arabic, was nearly as as long in perfectly uniting with half an ounce of diſtilled water, as that without the gum. This was perhaps owing to the latter piece being more reſinous; however, though on long ſtanding there was a ſmall ſediment, it immediately reunited a week after by agitation.

FIFTEEN grains of balſam capivi united very ſmoothly with half an ounce of diſtilled water, by the medium of three grains of gum arabic. Five grains of the gum were not ſo effectual with pump water.

BALSAM Peru ten drops, with gum arabic three grains, diſtilled water half an ounce, formed a neat white emulſion, but with common water a very unequal mixture.

GUM myrrh powdered, that there might be no difference in the ſeveral quantities uſed, half a ſcruple, diſſolved readily with gum arabic three grains, in both kinds of water,

water, and even mixed with them by longer trituration without any medium, but more eaſily with diſtilled than common ſpring water. Olibanum, maſtich, gum guaiacum, and galbanum may likewiſe be mixed with water by rubbing, without any gum arabic or egg.

THE ſpring water which was made uſe of was from my own pump, and is very aluminous.

IN the making of all the ſaline preparations, when any conſiderable quantities of water are uſed, diſtilled or pure rain, or river water is greatly to be preferred: For the calcareous, aluminous, and ſelenitical matter which ſo much abounds in moſt ſpring water, will render any ſalts diſſolved in it very impure. For ſeveral years before I came to reſide in this town, I had prepared *Magneſia Alba*, even ſuperior to that ſold by Mr. Glaſs; but on attempting to make it here, I was ſurpriſed and diſappointed to find it of greater ſpecific gravity, and more coarſe than uſual. I was for ſome time unable to account for the difference, as I had conducted the proceſs in every reſpect ſimilar to my former practice; but at laſt diſcovered it to depend wholly on the variation of the water: And I always obſerve the Magneſia to be light and pure, *cæteris paribus*, in proportion to the purity and ſoftneſs of the water I make uſe of. Nor will this be wondered at by any one who obſerves the quantity of calcareous earth and ſelenites, which is generally depoſited by the pump water of this town, when it has been boiled and has ſtood ſome time to cool.

THE ſolution of crude mercury with mucilage of gum arabic being ſo eaſily accompliſhed, and it being very diſagreeable to many patients, and to ſome almoſt impoſſible to ſwallow pills, boluſſes, or electuaries; I was induced to try whether calomel, cinnabar, and the other heavy and metalline bodies commonly adminiſtered

tered only under theſe forms, might not by the ſame means be rendered miſcible with water, ſo as to be given more agreeably in a liquid form.—I had indeed ſometimes ſeen injections made with calomel and gum arabic, but had not obſerved whether it ſuſpended the calomel ſo uniformly as to be given by the mouth.

I ACCORDINGLY rubbed ten grains of cinnabar of antimony and a ſcruple of gum arabic, with a ſufficient quantity of diſtilled water to form a mucilage, and added a drachm of ſimple ſyrup, and three drachms more of water.

THIS makes an agreeable little draught, and having ſtood about half an hour without depoſiting any ſediment, I added three drachms more of water to it, and notwithſtanding the mucilage was rendered ſo much more dilute, very little of the cinnabar ſubſided, even after it had ſtood ſome days.

STEEL ſimply prepared, and prepared tin were both mixed with water by their own weight of gum arabic, and remained ſuſpended, except a very ſmall portion of each, which was not reduced to a ſufficiently fine powder.

FIVE grains of calomel were mixed with two drachms of diſtilled water, and half a drachm of ſimple ſyrup, by means of five grains of gum arabic, which kept it ſufficiently ſuſpended: A double quantity of the gum preſerved the mixture uniform ſtill longer. In this form it will be much more eaſily given to children, than in ſyrups, conſerves, &c. as a great part of it is generally waſted, in forcing thoſe viſcid vehicles into them, and it may be joined with ſcammony and other reſinous purgatives by the ſame method, and of theſe perhaps the gum arabic would be the beſt corrector.

GUM arabic likewiſe greatly abates the diſagreeable taſte of the corroſive ſublimate,

mate, mixed with water inſtead of brandy; and (from the few trials I have made) ſits eaſier on the ſtomach, and will not be ſo apt to betray the patient by the ſmell of the brandy.

MR. PLENCK, who firſt inſtructed us in the method of mixing quick-ſilver with mucilage, obſerves, (and experience confirms the truth of it) that this preparation is not ſo apt to bring on a ſpitting as the *argent. viv.* mixed by any other medium, or as the ſaline and other mercurial preparations.—How far the theory by which he accounts for it may be juſt, is not of much importance, but it may perhaps be worth while to enquire whether it would not be equally effectual in preventing calomel, and the other preparations of mercury, from affecting the mouth.—If ſo, is it not improper where a ſalivation is intended, to give emulſions with gum arabic and other mucilaginous liquors for the patient's common drink, as by that means the ſpitting may be retarded?

tarded? And on the contrary, may it not be a uſeful medicine to diminiſh the diſcharge when too copious? (a)

BUT — *Ne ſutor ultra crepidam.* And though I am ſure your friendly candour will excuſe theſe trifling obſervations, which have occurred as I was writing, yet I fear I treſpaſs upon time which you would

(a) THE following caſe may in ſome meaſure ſerve to confirm the above obſervation.

A GENTLEMAN, always eaſily affected by mercurials, having taken about twenty-ſix grains of calomel in doſes from one to three grains, notwithſtanding he was purged every third day, was ſuddenly ſeized with a ſalivation. He ſpat plentifully, his breath was very fœtid, teeth looſe, and his gums, fauces, and the margin of his tongue greatly ulcerated and inflamed. He was directed to uſe the following gargle.

℞. *Gum. arab. ſemiunc. ſolve in aquæ font, bullient-ſelib. & adde mel. roſac. unc. unam. M. ft. gargar.*

AND to drink freely of a ptiſan prepared with *aq. hord. lib. ij. gum. arabic. unc. ij. nitr. pur. drachm. ij. ſacchar. alb. unc. j.*

HIS purgative was repeated the ſucceeding morning.

THE

would ſpend much more uſefully, than in peruſing theſe indigeſted thoughts of, dear Sir,

Your very obliged and humble Servant,

THOMAS HENRY.

THE next day his gums were leſs inflamed; but the ſloughs on his tongue, &c. were ſtill as foul; his ſpitting was much the ſame: he had drank about a pint of the ptiſan.—Some *ſpt. vitrioli* was added to the gargle.

FROM this day to the fourth, he was purged every day without effect—his ſalivation ſtill continued, his mouth was no better—he had neglected the mucilaginous drink—this evening he was perſuaded to drink about a pint of it which remained, and he had it repeated, and drank very freely of it that night.

ON the fifth morning the purgative was again repeated. Though it operated very little, yet the change was very ſurpriſing, his mouth was nearly well, and his ptyaliſm greatly decreaſed—the ptiſan was repeated, and on the ſixth day being quite well, he was permitted to go abroad.

SEE alſo Dr. Saunders's appendix to the ſecond edition of Mr. Plenck's Treatiſe, ſince publiſhed.

EXPERIMENT XIX.

It has been remarked by Professor Whytt, and many others, that different kinds of quick-lime impregnate water with different degrees of strength. This suggested to me that a diversity in the *menstruum*, may also considerably vary the qualities of the lime-water. And my conjecture has been confirmed by the ensuing experiments.

Equal quantities, viz. a quart, of distilled water, of boiled pump water grown cold, and of the same hard pump water unboiled, were severally added to half a pound of quick-lime. After an infusion of twenty-four hours, the waters were decanted off, and filtered through paper. Ten drops of syrup of violets struck a deep green with the lime water made with distilled water, a lighter one with that prepared with boiled water, and the lightest with the raw pump water. Sixty drops

drops of a ſolution of ſalt of tartar in diſtilled water, added to each lime water in the foregoing order, occaſioned the largeſt precipitation from the firſt, the next in degree from the ſecond, and the leaſt from the third. The taſtes of the different lime waters correſponded alſo with the above-mentioned teſts. For that made with diſtilled water was by far the moſt pungent, and yet the leaſt diſagreeable; whereas that prepared with raw pump water, was extremely harſh and nauſeous, without being proportionably impregnated with the acrimony of the quick-lime.

EXPERIMENT XX.

THREE fragments of human *calculi*, numbered for the ſake of diſtinction, 1, 2, 3, were immerſed in equal quantities of different lime waters; the firſt in lime water made with diſtilled water, the ſecond in lime water prepared with hard pump water, and the third in lime water made

made with the ſame hard pump water poured boiling hot upon the quick-lime. No. 1, was of a brown colour and hard texture, was ſmooth on one ſide and rough on the other, and weighed twenty-ſix grains and a half. No. 2, was a fragment of the ſame *calculus*, and weighed twenty five grains and a half. No. 3, a fragment of a different *calculus*, was of a looſer and more ſpongy texture than the former, and weighed twenty-ſeven grains. The phials which contained the *calculi* and four ounces by meaſure of lime water, were all nearly full, and cloſely corked up. After continuing the maceration eight days without heat, the *calculi* were taken out, carefully dried on filtering paper before a gentle fire, and then weighed. No. 1, had loſt a grain and a half, and was covered over in many parts of it with a ſoft, white, cretaceous matter. No. 2, had loſt only half a grain: Many little cryſtals ſhot from its ſurface. No. 3, had loſt a grain. But it ſhould be remembered, that this fragment was much ſofter

ſofter than the other two. The lime employed in this experiment was common ſtone quick-lime; that uſed in the former experiment, was brought out of Derbyſhire, and made of a ſpecies of marble containing a great many ſhells in its ſubſtance. I was not aware of the difference of the lime, till after my trials were compleated.

THESE two experiments, I think, ſatisfactorily prove, that ſoft water is a much more powerful diſſolvent of quick-lime, than hard water, *(a)* at the ſame time that it covers and meliorates the harſh taſte of that acrid ſubſtance. Where diſtilled water cannot conveniently be provided, rain water, freed by filtration from

(a) To aſcertain more fully this important point, I have ſince repeated the experiment above recited, by immerſing again the fragments of the ſame calculus, Nos. 1 and 2, in equal quantities of freſh lime water, prepared with diſtilled water, and with hard pump water. In twelve days, No. 1, was entirely reduced to a chalky powder, whilſt No. 2, preſerved its texture, to all appearance unchanged.

from its impurities, may with equal efficacy be ſubſtituted in its room. Had a different kind of lime been employed in the laſt experiment, or had the digeſtion been made in a ſand bath, it is probable the ſolvent power of each *menſtruum* would have been increaſed. The little pointed cryſtallizations, which were obſerved to ſhoot from the fragment of the *calculus* No. 2, remind me of a ſimilar appearance which occurred in one of the trials of the late Dr. Whytt, and which he informs us ſurpriſed him greatly. He aſcribes them to the ſea ſalt adhering, even after calcination, to the oyſter-ſhells which he employed. (a) But the Doctor muſt have been miſtaken in his explanation, as in the experiment juſt recited, common ſtone quick-lime alone was uſed, which cannot be ſuppoſed to contain any ſea ſalt. And the cryſtallizations were perceived only in that phial of lime water, which had been prepared with hard pump water.

(a) Whytt's Eſſay on Lime Water, 3d Edit. p. 74.

SEC-

SECTION III.

A COMPARATIVE VIEW OF THE DIFFERENT PROPERTIES OF SNOW WATER, RAIN WATER, SPRING WATER, &c.

SNOW WATER is ſaid by Mr. Boyle to be the lighteſt of all waters; and if received upon the tops of high mountains muſt, one ſhould conceive, be free from all foreign impregnation. And yet the ſame accurate chemiſt found on examination, that it is not entirely deſtitute of ſaltneſs. But notwithſtanding the ſuperior purity of ſnow water, I ſhould apprehend, that it is not the moſt wholeſome liquor for common drink, both from its extreme coldneſs, and becauſe its properties as a *menſtruum* are changed by the congelation it hath undergone. For freez-ing

ing decompoſes water, by ſeparating from it a conſiderable portion of air. And that this alters its qualities is evident from the following facts. 1. Water when freſh, diſſolves a larger quantity of ſalt, than when exhauſted of its air. 2. Water ſaturated with any ſalt, when placed *in vacuo* under the receiver of an air pump, will depoſit part of its ſolvend. 3. Snow water is obſerved not to boil greens or peaſe ſo well as common water. 4. The nitrous acid generates a much leſs degree of heat with ſnow water, than with common water. 5. Snow, mixed in a certain proportion with flour will, like eggs, render it when baked or boiled, perfectly light and adheſive. Hippocrates utterly condemns the uſe of ſnow or ice water, becauſe after congelation it never re-aſſumes its former nature; the clear, light, and ſweet part of it being diſſipated, whilſt the moſt turbid and heavy is left behind. And he adduces an experiment in ſupport of this reaſoning. Expoſe, ſays he, a veſſel containing a certain quantity

tity of water to the cold air in winter time, ſo as that it may be frozen hard; then bring it into a warm place, where it may thaw; and when the ice is diſſolved, meaſure the water again and you will find it evidently diminiſhed. But this loſs of bulk is not as Hippocrates ſuppoſes, to be aſcribed to the diſſipation of the thinner and finer parts of the water by congelation, but chiefly to the ſeparation of the air which it contained; and therefore his reaſon for condemning the uſe of ſnow water is founded on a falſe hypotheſis. This however does not invalidate his objection to it, which at firſt, in all probability, he deduced from experience, and afterwards attempted to explain and confirm, by what now appears to be miſtaken theory.

THE fertilizing effect of ſnow on the ground is univerſally known, and may in part ariſe from the covering which it affords to the earth, by which the aſcent of vapours is repreſſed, and a fermentation promoted

promoted in the ſoil. But I apprehend it depends not leſs upon the ſnow being deſtitute of air, ſo that like lime, when diſſolved and ſunk into the earth, it abſtracts air from the ſoil, occaſions an inteſtine motion in its particles, and thus pulveriſes them.

ICE WATER: What has been ſaid of ſnow water is equally applicable to ice water, except that its ſpecific gravity is greater, and that it is leſs free from ſaline impregnation, and conſequently ſtill leſs ſalubrious.

RAIN WATER, when collected in clean veſſels, at a diſtance from large towns, is light, ſoft, and wholeſome. But as it paſſes through the atmoſphere, which is a chaos of different exhalations from the animal, vegetable, and mineral kingdoms, it muſt waſh down ſome of thoſe floating, volatile particles, and be impregnated with them. Hence rain will differ in ſome ſlight degree, according

ing to the ſeaſon of the year, as well as the country in which it falls. That it contains a quantity of adventitious matter is evident from the curious experiments of M. Margraaf, from its tendency to putrefy, from the green weed which ſprings up on its ſurface, and from the mucilaginous or ropy ſubſtance which grows copiouſly on it, and which Boerhaave compares, on viewing it through a microſcope, to a grove of little muſhrooms. It is obſerved alſo, after ſtanding a while, to be full of the *ovula* of different animalcules; ſome of which may have been carried down with it, in its paſſage through the air, but the greater number are probably depoſited in it, during its ſtagnation. But although theſe circumſtances prove, that rain water is by no means an homogeneous fluid, or free from impurity, yet it is univerſally acknowledged to be the moſt ſalutary of all other kinds of water. And by percolation through ſand or ſtone, or by boiling and decanting, its foulneſs would in a great meaſure be ſeparated, and it would be rendered a grateful, potable, and very wholeſome liquor. Its levity is ſo great, that diſtilled rain water is not lighter than the natural, as Boerhaave affirms after weighing them in the hydroſtatical balance. Nor need we wonder at this, as the exhalation of aqueous vapours from the earth and ſea, is exactly analogous to diſtillation; if it be not an impropriety to compare the vaſt and ſtupendous operations of nature, with the trifling efforts of art. Hippocrates gives his teſtimony in favour of rain water, but directs that it ſhould be boiled or ſtrained; otherwiſe it has an ill ſmell, and occaſions a hoarſeneſs, and deep voice in thoſe who drink it. *(a)*

SPRING WATER: This muſt vary in its properties according to the nature of the ſoil, and different ſtrata of earth, through which it paſſes. The pureſt is that

(a) Hippoc. *de Aere, Aquis et Locis.*

that which flows, at no great depth, through a light gravel, or ſand. Dr. Hales mentions ſeveral ſprings remarkable for their levity, and freedom from calcareous impregnation. The water, conveyed by pipes to Hodſon in Hertfordſhire, which riſes from a gravel, and guſhes out of a fine white ſand, he informs us, left no incruſtation in a boiler, which had been uſed fifteen years. And that of Comb in Surrey, a hill the ſoil of which is gravel almoſt to the ſurface, is alſo uncommonly light, ſoft and free from all adventitious ingredients. As the ſprings iſſue from the brow of the hill, out of the gravel, the Doctor juſtly obſerves, that the water muſt partake greatly of the nature of rain water; ſince the dew and rain which fall on that hill, receive probably no other alteration from percolating through the gravel, than that of being rendered more pure and free from foulneſs. *(a)* Hippocrates lays a

 great

(a) Vid. Statical Eſſays, Vol. 2. p. 242.

great ſtreſs upon the choice of ſprings, which have an eaſtern aſpect. Such waters, he ſays, are chiefly to be commended, that guſh out towards the riſing of the ſun; becauſe they are clearer, lighter, and of a better ſmell than others. But I apprehend there is no foundation for this opinion: For water which flows through clay, marle, black mould, or beds of minerals, will be equally hard and unwholeſome in whatever expoſure it firſt burſts out. The purity and ſalubrity of it may however, with ſufficient accuracy be aſcertained, by its levity, tranſparency, and perfect inſipidity; by its mingling uniformly with ſoap, and boiling pulſe tender. And theſe are common teſts, which it is in the power of every one to apply.

River Water: This is generally much ſofter, and better adapted to œconomical uſes than moſt ſpring water. For though rivers proceed originally from ſprings,

ſprings, yet by their rapid motion,(a) and by being expoſed during a long courſe, to the influence of the ſun and air, the earthy and metallic ſalts which they contain are in part decompoſed, the volatile acid flies off, and the terreſtrial or ochery particles with which it was combined, become inſoluble and are precipitated. To this it may be added, that rivers are alſo rendered ſofter by the vaſt quantity of rain water, which paſſing along the ſurface of the earth, is immediately conveyed into their channels. But all rivers carry with them, a great deal of mud, filth, and other impurities. And when they flow near large, populous, and manufacturing towns, they become the receptacles of all the common ſewers, and are impregnated with an heterogene-

(a) THE Rhine and the Rhone, which flow from the Alps, whilſt they preſerve the rapidity of their courſe, are obſerved to be light and pure. The difference betwixt the Rhine and the Maine, is obvious to thoſe who navigate theſe rivers: For the barges which ſail from the latter into the former, ſink conſiderably deeper in the one, than in the other.

Lucas, Vol. 1. p. 35.

ous mixture of coperas, alum, ſoap lyes, logwood, and the refuſe of a thouſand other ſubſtances, employed in different arts. In this ſtate, river water is certainly unfit for the common purpoſes of life. And yet if it be ſuffered to remain a while at reſt, all the feculencies will ſubſide, and the water will become ſufficiently pure, grateful, and potable.

STAGNANT WATERS: Theſe of all others are the moſt impure and inſalubrious. Hippocrates aſſerts that they enlarge and obſtruct the ſpleen; and his obſervation is almoſt daily confirmed, by the diſſection of thoſe who die of the ſcurvy; a diſeaſe which putrid, ſtagnant water hath a powerful tendency to produce. Dr. Hoffman, by means of a glaſs waterpoiſe divided by lines, examined hydroſtatically ſeveral different kinds of water. Rain water he found to be the lighteſt; river water was one line heavier; the water commonly uſed at Hall, in Saxony, was heavier by two lines; the ſpring water of the ſame

ſame place was four lines heavier; that of a particular ſpring was ſix lines heavier; and water which had been long kept in an open veſſel, in a cellar, was ſix lines and a half; but ſtagnant water, drawn out of the town ditch at Hall, was ſeven lines heavier than rain water. (a)

I SHALL conclude this Eſſay with the following obſervations of Celſus, which in many reſpects coincide with what has been advanced. *Aqua leviſſima pluviatilis eſt; deinde fontana, tum ex flumine, tum ex puteo; poſt hæc ex nive aut glacie; gravior his ex lacu; graviſſima ex palude. Facilis etiam et neceſſaria cognitio eſt naturam ejus requirentibus. Nam levis pondere apparet, & ex his quæ pondere pares ſunt, eo melior quæque eſt, quo celerius et caleſit & frigeſcit, quoque celerius ex ea legumina percoquuntur.* (b)

(a) *Vid.* Hoffman Obſ. Chem. p. 140.
(b) Celſus Lib. 2. Cap. 18.

A REVIEW OF THE PRINCIPAL FACTS ASCERTAINED BY THE PRECEDING EXPERIMENTS.

1. THE Mancheſter pump water is in general very hard and impure. It is impregnated with a large quantity of ſelenite, and contains alſo no inconſiderable proportion of alum.

2. THE hardeſt water will become ſoft and miſcible with ſoap, by the addition of ſalt of tartar. But ſuch a quantity of the vegetable alkali is required, to produce this effect on the Mancheſter pump water, as renders it offenſive to the palate, and unfit for common uſe.

3. HARD water is conſiderably ſoftened by boiling. For though heat generally increaſes the diſſolving power of any *menſtruum*,

menſtruum, at the ſame time it tends, in many inſtances, to deſtroy the texture, and diſunite the component parts of the ſolvend. Thus the groſſer ſalts contained in hard water are decompoſed by the boiling heat; the volatile vitriolic or muriatic acids fly off, leaving behind them an indiſſoluble, petrefying earth, which ſubſides to the bottom, and incruſts the veſſel. But the coction ſhould be continued fifteen or twenty minutes, to produce its full effect. The water ſhould then be ſuffered to remain a few hours expoſed to the atmoſphere, to recover its due proportion of air before it be uſed. For the loſs of this air by boiling, alters the properties of water, and probably may render it leſs ſalutary.

4. HARD water is ſoftened by being filtered through ſtone. And if it were firſt boiled a ſufficient length of time, and then filtered, it would be rendered tolerably pure, potable, and ſalutary, and at the

the ſame time much better adapted to a variety of culinary uſes.

5. Mr. Boyle aſſerts, that ſome pump waters, by expoſure to the ſun and air for a few days, will become ſoft enough to be miſcible with ſoap. But this is not the caſe with the hard water of Mancheſter.

6. Neither malt nor tea produce any ſoftening effect, on the hard water in which they are infuſed. Nor does fermentation improve or alter its nature. So that the wholeſomeneſs of malt liquors, muſt greatly depend upon the purity of the water, which is employed in their preparation.

7. Bricks harden the ſofteſt water, and give it an aluminous impregnation. The practice of lining wells with them, which is common in many places, is therefore very improper. Free-ſtone communicates no pernicious qualities to water.

8. Though

8. THOUGH by the tables of elective attractions it appears, that the acid of vitriol hath a ſtronger affinity to lead, than to the earth of alum, yet this metal does not appear by experiment, to be ſoluble in aluminous waters. But perhaps the volatile tincture of ſulphur may not, in every inſtance, be a certain criterion of the preſence of lead, as green vitriol is not of the aſtringency of vegetables. And a proportion of this poiſonous mineral, too minute to be diſcovered by any chemical examination, may in irritable habits, and under certain delicate circumſtances, prove highly injurious to health.

9. SOFT water, and eſpecially diſtilled water, acts far more powerfully as a *menſtruum* on vegetable bitters and aſtringents, than hard pump water. And it diſſolves reſinous bodies without any medium, or at leaſt with a much ſmaller proportion of mucilage of gum arabic, than is commonly employed.

10. HARD,

10. HARD, aluminous waters are likely to ſucceed beſt in the dying of black, red, and other colours, which require aſtringency, and alſo in the preparation of ink.

11. SOFT water is a much more powerful diſſolvent of quick-lime, than hard water; at the ſame time that it covers and improves the harſh taſte of that acrid ſubſtance. The fragment of a human *calculus* was entirely reduced to a chalky powder, by being immerſed twelve days in lime-water, prepared with diſtilled water; whereas another fragment of the ſame *calculus* ſuffered no viſible change in its texture, by being macerated an equal length of time in lime-water, made with common pump water.

12. IN nephritic caſes, diſtilled water would be a good ſubſtitute for Malvern-water; for it is a powerful ſolvent of the human *calculus*.

ON

ON THE

DISADVANTAGES

OF

INOCULATING CHILDREN

IN

EARLY INFANCY.

THE SECOND EDITION, REVISED AND ENLARGED.

Non quæ mihi suggessit phantasiæ imaginatricis temeritas, sed quæ phænomena practica edocuere.

SYDENHAM.

ON THE

DISADVANTAGES

OF

INOCULATING CHILDREN

IN EARLY INFANCY.

THE advantages arising from inoculation are now so universally acknowledged, that arguments in support of it seem to be entirely unnecessary. The rapid progress it hath made, affords the strongest presumption in favour of its safety and utility; and the well-attested accounts which we every day read, of the success with which it is practised, justly remove every prejudice against it, whether political or religious. The patrons of inoculation therefore, have nothing to fear from its avowed enemies, if if any ſuch there be; but they have the utmoſt reaſon to guard againſt the miſtaken zeal of its friends, which may prove perhaps more dangerous to its real intereſt, than oppoſition itſelf. Credulity, faſhion, the love of novelty, and a propenſity to ruſh from one extreme to another, are principles which have too much influence on the generality of mankind. And how unfavourable theſe have been to the advancement and perpetuity of improvements, might be demonſtrated by numerous examples. That the artificial method of communicating the ſmall-pox, ſo happily introduced amongſt us, may not hereafter be added to this diſgraceful liſt, every ſincere advocate for it, ſhould exert his warmeſt endeavours to diſcourage the wanton levity, with which it is at preſent in many places adopted. For the indiſcriminate uſe of remedies, exceſs in the cooling regimen, and a total diſregard to age, temperament, and habit of body, cannot fail in the iſſue to injure the reputation, and check the progreſs of one

of

of the moſt important diſcoveries in the whole circle of phyſic.

In the third volume of the Medical Observations and Inquiries, Doctor Maty, a learned and ingenious Phyſician in London, hath inſerted an Eſſay on the advantages of very early inoculation. He propoſes that people ſhould be induced by perſuaſion, and by other encouragements if neceſſary, to inoculate their children as ſoon as poſſible after their birth. And this he conſiders as the *maximum*, to which the art of inoculation can be brought, both with reſpect to individuals, and to the public. But the Doctor's reaſoning in ſupport of his hypotheſis, appears to me to be more ingenious and plauſible, than ſolid and ſatisfactory. And I apprehend the practice which he recommends, would conſiderably diminiſh the benefits ariſing from inoculation, and would be of dangerous and fatal conſequence to mankind. I ſhall endeavour therefore to point out the disadvantages which would attend the ingraftment of the small-pox on new-born children; and shall also make some strictures on Dr. MATY's arguments in favour of it.

1. THE number of diseases to which infants are incident, render them unfit subjects for inoculation. HIPPOCRATES, two thousand years ago remarked, *Ætatibus morbosissimi sunt juniores*. And when we consider the great and sudden changes, both external and internal, which they undergo at birth; the laxity and wonderful delicacy of their frame, and their extreme irritability perhaps depending upon it; the copiousness of the glandular secretions, with the difficulty of preserving that equilibrium, the least deviation from which affects them; it is matter of real astonishment, that life itself can be supported, under a series of such apparently unfavourable circumstances. Scarcely hath the little stranger been ushered into the world, but he discovers signs of indisposition,

indiſpoſition, by his reſtleſſneſs, anxiety, crying, and vomiting, by the ſwelling of his belly, and ſometimes by convulſions. Theſe ſymptoms ariſe from the load of *meconium* with which the ſtomach and bowels are oppreſſed, and generally ceaſe when thoſe organs have been gently evacuated. The jaundice next ſucceeds, and is ſometimes complicated with a very acrimonious ſtate of the fluids, as appears by the eruption of little red puſtules, with which the ſkin is every where loaded. The thruſh, watery gripes, and convulſions obſerve no regular order of time, but attack moſt infants, either ſingly or collectively, according as they are more or leſs obnoxious to the cauſes which produce them. The quick growth of children in the firſt period after birth, is likewiſe a ſource of numerous ailments; notwithſtanding the proviſion which nature hath made, to guard againſt the inconveniences reſulting from it, by the laxity of the glandular ſyſtem. The ſudden enlargement of the fœtus, in the womb of the mother is truly ſurpriſing. Dr. HARVEY relates, that in the deer kind, he obſerved the *punctum ſaliens*, on the 19th or 20th of November. On the 21ſt he ſaw the *vermiculus* or embryo of the animal; and on the 27th the fœtus was ſo perfect, that the male might be diſtinguiſhed from the female, the feet were formed, and the hoofs were cloven. This rapid growth muſt be aſcribed to the ſoft and yielding ſtructure of the fœtus, to the plenty of nutrition it receives, to its exemption from all diſcharges, and to the proportionably ſtrong action of its little heart. And as moſt of theſe cauſes continue to exert their influence after birth, though in a leſs degree, the increment of the young animal proceeds apace, and redundancies are formed, which in a healthy ſtate are carried off by one or other of the glandular excretions. But a deficiency or exceſs in any of theſe, neceſſarily produce diſeaſes. And in ſuch feeble, delicate, and irritable ſubjects, the equilibrium cannot long be preſerved. If they

are

are defective, all the complaints which arise from plenitude ensue; the child grows feverish, dull, and comatose; his stomach is disordered, his bowels are oppressed with wind, and if his belly be constipated he falls into convulsions. On the other hand, if they are excessive, a *diarrhœa* is produced, *aphthæ* and severe gripes succeed, and the violent irritation seldom fails to occasion epileptic fits. From this short view of the first period of infancy, I think it must appear evident, that inoculation is ill adapted to that tender season of life. Nature, feeble and irritable as she then is, can scarcely struggle with the diseases to which she is ordinarily exposed. It is therefore equally cruel and unjust to add to the number with which she is already oppressed. For it is demonstrable from the bills of mortality, that two thirds of all who are born, live not to be two years old; and I think it is more than probable, that a considerable proportion of these, die under the age of six weeks.

2. The fears and anxiety of the mother, excited at a time when her ſtrength hath been exhauſted by the pains of labour, and when every uneaſy impreſſion ſhould be cautiouſly avoided, cannot fail to injure her milk. And this is a powerful objection to the early ingraftment of infants. If a hired nurſe be employed, her milk may diſagree with the child, ſhe may fall into ſome diſeaſe during the time of inoculation, may be guilty of exceſs in eating or drinking, or may be under the influence of violent paſſions; each of which will aggravate the ſymptoms, and increaſe the danger of the artificial diſtemper, under which the infant labours. (a)

3. It

(a) Infantes ex aſſumpto lacte nutricis, quæ brevi ante ira vel terrore perculſa fuit, in graviſſima pathemata, convulſiva, epileptica, & ſæviſſima alvi tormina incidant.

Hoffman. Op. Vol. 1. p. 196.

A child, whoſe mother was its nurſe, became feveriſh on the third day of eruption, which cauſed violent anxiety in the mother, a raſh with coſtive belly, was then obſerved, and the child died on the ſecond day after it.

Monro's Acct. of Inoc. in Scot. p. 25.

A nurse

3. It hath been obſerved by a very able and experienced practitioner, (a) that young children have uſually a larger ſhare of puſtules from inoculation, than thoſe who are a little farther advanced in life: And that from this circumſtance ſo many have died, as to diſcourage the practice of ingrafting the ſmall pox on ſuch delicate ſubjects. This fact is not eaſy to be explained. Whether the greater irritability of infants ſubjects them to be more affected with the variolous *miaſma*, than children of two or three years old; or whether the larger eruption, to which they are liable, be owing to the proportionably greater quantity of their fluids,

 I will

A nurse of an inoculated child who died, was diſcovered to have drank immoderately of malt liquor, during the proceſs of inoculation.

Monro's Acc. of Inoc. in Scot p. 33.

The nurſe of an inoculated child who died, was ſuſpected to have been tainted with the Lues venerea, by her huſband, who was afterwards diſcovered to have had the diſeaſe, and at the time ſhe was nurſing the child.

Monro's Acc. of Inoc. in Scot. p. 33.

(a) Baron Dimsdale.

I will not presume to determine. Both causes may possibly conspire to produce this effect; the former by exciting a quicker, and increased contraction of the heart and vascular system; the latter by affording a more copious *pabulum* for the variolous ferment. By the same principles we may perhaps account for the greater virulence of the *lues venerea*, in infancy, than in the more advanced stages of life.

4. A CONSIDERABLE number of those who die of the natural disease, before the expulsion of the variolous eruption, are infants or very young children. (a) This does not arise, as Dr. KIRKPATRICK supposes, from the extreme weakness of the *vis vitæ* of infants; for the contraction of their hearts is proportionably stronger than in adults, as the quickness of their growth evinces; but from the high degree of irritability with which their nervous

(a) KIRKPATRICK's Analysis.

vous ſyſtem is endued. Hence the convulſive paroxyſms, which often precede the appearance of the puſtules, and which, though regarded by SYDENHAM as no unfavourable ſigns, are always alarming, and when they happen to very young infants, are frequently fatal.

5. IF ſuch a number of puſtules ſhould break out in the mouth or throat as to obſtruct ſuction, the diſeaſe, in all probability, would prove fatal. Even a few pocks in thoſe parts are highly troubleſome and dangerous to infants; for beſides the pain and reſtleſſneſs which they produce, they often terminate in ill conditioned ulcers.*(a)*

6. THOSE who are affected with cutaneous diſeaſes, have been generally regarded as unfavourable ſubjects of inoculation. *(b)* Infancy, therefore, which is ſeldom unattended with eruptions on the ſkin,

(a) Vid. SCHULTS on Inoculation.

(b) DR. JURIN's Account of Inoculation.

ſkin, muſt be an improper period for receiving the ſmall pox by ingraftment.

7. THE thickneſs of the teguments of infants, which ariſes from the quantity of fluids interpoſed between their fibres, by which the ſkin is rendered ſoft and œdematous to the touch, and their perſpiring leſs than children who are capable of uſing exerciſe, are further objections to very early inoculation.

8. BUT the moſt forcible argument againſt this practice, is deduced from the ill-ſucceſs 'which hath attended infant inoculation in general. For it appears by Dr. JURINS' account of the progreſs of inoculation in Great-Britain from 1721 to 1726, and by Dr. SCHEUCHZER's continuation of it to 1728, that of fifty eight children under two years old, who received the ſmall-pox by ingraftment, ſix died; whereas of two hundred and twenty one, inoculated between the ages of two and five, only three died.

HAVING

HAVING thus pointed out ſome of the principal objections to the early inoculation of infants, I ſhall make a few remarks on Dr. MATY's ingenious Eſſay in favour of it. After enumerating the advantages which infancy has with regard to the ſmall-pox, the Doctor ſums up the whole by ſaying: "If there is a period "in which the machine is in a perfect "ſtate, it certainly is immediately before "it begins to be ſpoiled, or at the firſt "period after nativity." *(a)* This aſſertion, I apprehend, is repugnant to reaſon, anatomy, and experience. It ſeems to be a general law of nature, that all organiſed bodies ſhould advance by progreſſive ſtages to their acme or ſtate of perfection; and ſhould then decline by the ſame regular gradation. A plant when it firſt ſprings out of the ground is frail and tender, by degrees the ſtem thickens, the leaves expand themſelves, the juices are concocted, the flower opens, the ſeed is formed, ripened, and ſhed; and

(a) Medical Obſervations, Vol. 3. p. 290.

and when the office aſſigned it by the ſovereign Creator is thus accompliſhed, it droops, withers, and falls into decay. The animal world furniſhes ſtill more ſtriking proofs of the truth of this obſervation. And I know nothing which contributes more to the beauty and harmony of the univerſe, or affords a more admirable diſplay of the wiſdom of its great Author, than the order and uniformity with which theſe ſucceſſive changes are carried on, amongſt the different claſſes of beings.

From the reſearches of anatomiſts into the ſtructure of the human body, it is evident that our machine in infancy is comparatively extremely imperfect, that its parts are diſproportioned, and its organs incapable of thoſe functions, which they are deſtined in future life to perform. The head of a new-born child, bears a much larger proportion to the bulk of his body, than that of an adult; the former being as one to three, the latter only as one

one to eight. And this joined to the remarkable laxity of the fibres in infancy, is the reason perhaps of the excessive irritability with which the body is then endued, and which lays a foundation for numerous diseases. The Liver and Pancreas are so immensely distended, as to fill up almost the whole cavity of the abdomen; and the copiousness of their secretions is equal to their bulk. The bile, cystic and hepatic, is almost insipid, and so inert that it is incapable either of promoting digestion, or of neutralizing those acidities, which the weakness of the stomachs, and the acescency of the food of infants, generate in the *primæ viæ*. Hence probably arise the crudities, flatulency, gripes, aphthæ, and convulsions, to which children, at that tender age, are peculiarly exposed. The heart, with respect to the vascular system, is both stronger and more bulky in infancy than in after life. *(a)* By this means the blood is propelled

(a) By the curious tables of Dr. Bryan Robinson, it appears, that the weight of the heart with respect to the weight

pelled with greater force; and as the arteries at that period have leſs firmneſs and denſity than the veins, as appears by Sir CLIFTON WINTRINGHAM's experiments, they are then moſt yielding and diſtenſile. And both theſe cauſes equally conſpire to promote and quicken the growth of the young animal. But wiſe and neceſſary as this proviſion of nature is, it unavoidably expoſes the infant to all the dangers which ariſe from a plethora, and muſt be conſidered as a preſent imperfection, however well adapted it may be to thoſe progreſſive changes, which advance him from childhood to maturity. For by degrees the heart abates of its proportional force, and the arteries acquire their greateſt amplitude. At this period the moving

weight of the body, is greater in a child than in a man, in the proportion of three to two: that the quantity of blood which flows through the heart in a given time is greater in children than in grown bodies, in the proportion of twenty to ſeven, which is the proportion of their pulſes in a minute: and that the velocity of the blood is greater in a child than a man, in the proportion of eighty to ſeven.

moving powers of the machine are equally balanced, and the body ſeems to enjoy for a while a ſtate of reſt. But the delicate equilibrium cannot long be maintained: The heart grows feeble and languid, the arteries gradually contract themſelves, a venous plenitude enſues, and old age cloſes the ſcene.

BUT analogy may deceive us, and the obſervations of anatomiſts may be doubtful; experience however carries conviction along with it, and inconteſtibly demonſtrates, that the human body, contrary to the aſſertion of Dr. MATY, is moſt imperfect in the firſt period after nativity. For it is univerſally acknowledged, that infancy is liable to a much greater variety of maladies than any other ſtage of life. This can ariſe only from the extreme delicacy of the ſtructure, and diſproportion of the parts of new-born children; and both the cauſe and effect, in this inſtance, are marks of frailty and imperfection.

"CONVUL-

" CONVULSIONS in young babes, ſays " Dr. MATY, ſeem to be, not ſo much " a diſeaſe, as an indication of ſome diſ- " order in the bowels, or the effort of " nature to expel ſome enemy." *(a)* The obſervation is in general juſt, for I believe the true idiopathic convulſions happen very rarely. But though ſomewhat leſs alarming on this account, theſe fits are always attended, in ſuch feeble and delicate ſubjects with imminent danger. Many it is well known have expired under them; while others, who have ſtruggled through with great difficulty, have been ſo debilitated, and their faculties ſo impaired, that the effects have been perceptible during the remaining part of their lives. *(b)* The convulſions about the time of the eruption, and ſubſiding of the inoculated ſmall-pox, ſays Dr. Monro, are the moſt frequent bad ſymptom in this diſeaſe; and by them more of thoſe in the

(a) Medical Obſervations, Vol. 3. p. 292.

(b) DIMSDALE on Inoculation.

the column of dead, loſt their lives, than by any other cauſe. *(a)*

"THAT diſpoſition in the inteſtinal "tube to excoriate, which ariſes from "the too great aceſcency of milk or ve-"getable aliments, is eaſily corrected by "magneſia, lime-water, oil, and by "ſmall quantities of broth or other ani-"mal food." *(b)* The remedies which Dr. MATY hath here pointed out, are very judicious and proper; but their effects are much more uncertain than he ſeems to apprehend. The ailments of children are generally very complicated, and the indications of cure are often obſcure and doubtful. In their irritable bodies, one ſymptom frequently brings on a variety of others, ſometimes connected with the original one, at other times, to all appearance totally diſſimilar. And theſe ſymptoms of ſymptoms,

 as

(a) Monro's Account of Inoculation in Scotland, p. 25.
(b) Medical Obſervations, Vol. 3. p. 293.

as they are termed, do not always ceaſe, when the cauſe which firſt produced them is removed. This every phyſician experiences, who is converſant with the diſeaſes of infants; and it neceſſarily occaſions, in his treatment of them, ſome degree of difficulty and confuſion.

From the liſts of Dr. Jurin, and Dr. Scheuchzer, Dr. Maty finds that nine out of two hundred and ſeventy-three, i. e. one out of thirty, inoculated under five years of age, died between the years 1721, and 1728. But if the doctor had confined himſelf, as he ought to have done, to the liſt of thoſe who died by inoculation under one year old, he would have found the proportion to be vaſtly greater, viz. no leſs than one in twelve. But as even one in thirty is a great mortality, and as the operation in grown people, during that period, appears to have carried off only one in fifty; Dr. M. endeavours to obviate this objection in the following manner: "As ſo "many

"many more children under five years, "die of different diſorders, than at any "other age, it is more than probable "that ſeveral, perhaps moſt of theſe "nine would have died, though they "had not been inoculated." (a) But though the Doctor has given ſome good reaſons for preſuming upon this probability, I would aſk him where is the juſtice or propriety of ingrafting the ſmall-pox at a period when, from the inſtances he himſelf adduces, the riſque appears to be ſo great of other dangerous, and fatal diſtempers acceding to it? For ſlightly as this artificial diſeaſe is now regarded, it is of itſelf ſufficient for the powers of nature to ſtruggle with in early infancy.

THE ſecond part of Dr. MATY's eſſay, diſplays the political advantages, which would accrue from the early inoculation of infants. But if it be evident from what has been advanced, that the practice he

(a) Medical Obſervations, Vol. 3. p. 295.

recommends, is prejudicial to individuals, it will require no arguments to prove that it muſt be equally ſo to the public. The abſurd cuſtom of ſeparating, in the bills of mortality, the ages of thoſe who die, from the diſeaſes by which they are carried off, renders it impoſſible to aſcertain with preciſion, the riſque of the natural ſmall-pox, which is incurred by delaying inoculation. But from my own experience, as well as from the obſervations of the moſt intelligent of my medical friends, I ſhould conclude this riſque to be very trifling; and that the ſmall-pox is a diſtemper to which children, in the firſt period of life, are rarely liable. For at that tender age they are neither in the way of infection, nor are they much diſpoſed to receive it. Dr. Monro informs us, that of twelve infants, inoculated within a fortnight after their birth, not one had the variolous eruption.*(a)*

To

(a) Monro on Inoculation, p. 25.

To conclude: Though infants are leſs proper ſubjects for receiving the ſmall-pox by ingraftment, than children a little further advanced in life, yet it muſt be confeſſed, that ſuch circumſtances may occur, as to render the inoculation of them highly expedient and adviſeable. In ſuch caſes however, I think the age of two or three months, is preferable to the period which Dr. Maty recommends. For it will then be too early to apprehend any diſturbance from dentition; and yet the child will have ſurmounted ſome of the diſeaſes, peculiar to the firſt ſtage of its exiſtence. The chylopoietic organs will alſo by that time have been ſo ſtrengthened by exerciſe and habit, as to diſcharge their functions with ſome degree of regularity. But the fitteſt ſeaſon for inoculation ſeems to be, between the age of two and four in healthy children, and of three and ſix in thoſe who are extremely tender and delicate. The powers of nature are then ſufficiently vigorous; perſpiration is free and copious; the irritability of the body is greatly diminiſhed; the viſcera are ſound and unobſtructed; the mind though active and lively, is not diſturbed by violent emotions; the teguments are properly extenuated; and the fibres are neither too tenſe, nor too lax for the variolous eruption. To theſe important advantages may be added, that at this age the child is both a proper ſubject for preparatory medicines, and for ſuch as may be deemed neceſſary during the courſe of the diſtemper. It is no wonder therefore, that the practice of inoculation is attended with moſt ſucceſs at this period. And it is ſeriouſly to be lamented, that the precious opportunity ſhould ever be neglected.

ON

ON THE EFFICACY OF EXTERNAL APPLICATIONS IN THE ULCEROUS SORE THROAT.

*Ad utilitatem Vitæ omnia consilia factaq;
nostra dirigenda sunt.*

TACITUS.

ON THE EFFICACY OF

EXTERNAL APPLICATIONS

IN THE

ANGINA MALIGNA,

OR,

ULCEROUS SORE THROAT.

THE ANGINA MALIGNA is for the moſt part ſo rapid in its progreſs, that it requires all the aſſiſtance of art to counteract its malignity, and to prevent its fatal termination: And when children are attacked with it, we are often reduced to the moſt diſtreſſing perplexity from the difficulty of perſuading, or the danger and impoſſibility of forcing them to uſe thoſe means which are neceſſary for their relief. It has been my misfortune lately to attend ſeveral ſuch froward patients, whoſe whofe cafes, independent on their perverfenefs, afforded the moft unfavourable prognoftics, and obliged me to depend entirely on external applications. The following method of cure I have hitherto fuccefsfully purfued.

A PLASTER compofed of *Emplaft. Stomach.* or *Emplaft. è Cymino p. ij. Emp. Vefic. p. j. Camph. S. V. R. trit.* ℥*ifs*, is directed to be applied to the nape of the neck, and a cataplafm of *Cort. Peruv. & Flor. Chamœm.* boiled in vinegar, with the addition of two drachms of camphor, to be laid acrofs the throat, and renewed every four hours. Sometimes inftead of this cataplafm, a flannel moiftened with equal parts of camphorated fpirit of wine and vinegar is recommended, which is highly refrefhing and grateful to the patient.

A PEDILUVIUM confifting of the abovementioned ingredients, viz. bark and chamomile flowers, boiled in vinegar and water

water, is prefcribed to be ufed three or four times in a day. When the weaknefs of the patient renders him unable to fit with his feet in the bath, cloths lightly wrung out of the decoction are ordered to be wrapped round his legs and thighs.

To medicate the air, both for the benefit of the patient and of his attendants, fuch a compofition as Dr. Huxham recommends, viz. chamomile flowers, rofemary and myrrh with vinegar, is advifed to be kept boiling over the lamp of a teakettle, fo that the vapour, which is by no means difagreeable, may be diffufed through the room; and the lamp is fometimes placed near the bedfide of the fick perfon, that he may infpire the antifeptic fteams more copioufly.

My reafon for prefcribing a bliftering plafter under the form above directed, is becaufe I have found by experience, that the fkin in this diforder is very eafily inflamed and veficated; and that a fufficiently

ently copious diſcharge of ſerum is procured by this compoſition, which at the ſame time coincides with the general indication of correcting putridity. And I muſt here beg leave to remark, that early bliſtering in the *angina maligna* has a peculiarly good effect; though I am no advocate in general for the application of veſicatories, in the beginning of fevers.

THE cataplaſm ſeems to me, to anſwer ſeveral uſeful purpoſes: It tends to ſoften and relax the glands of the neck, which are often tumefied in this diſorder; it continually exhales an antiſeptic vapour, which is drawn into the mouth and fauces at every inſpiration; and no inconſiderable portion of it is carried into the ſyſtem by abſorption. And it appears not improbable, from the common methods of preventing putrefaction in animal fleſh, that ſome part of it may paſs to the ſeat of the diſeaſe, by penetrating through the interſtices of the muſcular fibres,

fibres, when the cellular membrane is not loaded with fat.

The uſe of the *pediluvium* in every ſpecies of fever is acknowledged to be highly ſerviceable, and is peculiarly ſo in this diſorder, in which the ſkin is hot and dry, and the efflorescence on the ſurface of the body apt to diſappear from the ſlighteſt cauſes, producing an aggravation of all the ſymptoms. Beſides its relaxing and antiſpaſmodic effects, it tends to bring on a ſwelling of the feet, which I have ſometimes obſerved, to be ſo beneficial to the patient, as almoſt inclined me to think it a critical derivation. By the addition of bark, chamomile flowers, and vinegar, the *pediluvium* is rendered powerfully antiſeptic, without any diminution of its other effects. An ingenious writer has propoſed a method of conveying a very large portion of nitre into the body, as a corrector of putrefaction; but in the ſore throat, and every putrid diſeaſe, could ſuch a quantity be intro-

introduced into the courſe of the circulation, it would, I apprehend, diſappoint our expectations, and by weakening the *vis vitæ* increaſe the ſeptic ferment.

THESE means aſſiduouſly purſued, have hitherto ſucceeded to my wiſhes, though I ſhould not chuſe to truſt to them alone when other remedies could be employed. However ſuch is my confidence in their efficacy, that I would never fail to recommend them, along with frequent gargling, and the internal uſe of the *cortex*, wine, &c.

AN eminent practitioner has very judiciouſly recommended, in the firſt ſtage of the diſorder, the waſhing of the ſtomach with a gentle emetic. This advice I have generally purſued, and have always obſerved, that it mitigated the violence of the ſymptoms, and in ſome inſtances has entirely removed the diſeaſe. The efficacy of emetics in this diſtemper is not to be aſcribed ſolely to the evacuation

cuation which they produce of the contents of the ſtomach, but to their unloading the glands of the throat, promoting an equal circulation, and increaſing perſpiration.

I DO not recollect that any authors have taken notice of a ſymptom, which has not unfrequently attended the ſore throat, as it has appeared in this neighbourhood, I mean a very fœtid, ichorous diſcharge from the ears. In the beginning of the preſent ſummer (1770) this ſymptom occurred only in the worſt caſes, and ſuch as generally proved fatal: I have lately obſerved it ſeveral times when the patient has recovered; but indurated parotids, and deafneſs have enſued.

I HAVE met with ſeveral caſes in which all the ſymptoms of the *angina maligna* have appeared, excepting the ulcers of the throat: Nor could there be any doubt concerning the nature of the diſeaſe, as the patients had been expoſed to the infection

infection of it. These instances, I apprehend, incontestibly prove the ulcerous sore throat to be a distemper of the whole habit, and not almost entirely a local affection, as may be inferred to be the opinion of a very learned and eminent Physician, whose writings contain a treasure of medical knowledge, from his laying *the chief stress of the cure on gargling*.

ALTHOUGH we should be cautious in the use of the vegetable acids, from their tendency to renew or increase the *diarrhœa*, yet the mineral acids are not liable to this objection, and I think may be administered with great advantage: I frequently direct the dulcified spirit of nitre to be given freely in an infusion of red rose leaves, mixed with port wine. It is cordial, antiseptic, and gently diaphoretic, and thus answers several very important indications.

A GENERAL

INDEX.

I N D E X.

B.

 force

C.

D.

L.

M.

Maty,

Pediluvium,

INDEX.

Salts,

S.

T.

warm

V.

W.

Yellow

INDEX.

Y.

THE END.

ERRATA.

Page 11, line 11, for Potterfield read Porterfield.
Page 30, line 9, for epedemic read epidemic.
Page 98, line 18, for floculent read flocculent.
Page 124, line 12, after ſolution read of.
Page 135, line 3 of the note, for proabbly read probably.
Page 143, line 8, for œger read æger.
Page 147, line 7, for ilico read illico.
Page 226, line 5, for begun read began.
Page 241, line 11, for alternative read alternate.
Page 252, line 20, for broke read broken.
Page 260, line 2 of the note, for ſacharine read ſaccharine.
Page 260, line 9, for realy read really.
Page 294, twice, for ſacharum read ſaccharum.
Page 306, line 7, for Swieton read Swieten.
Page 307, line 15, for therefote read therefore.
Page 308, line 22, for ſacharum read ſaccharum.
Page 317, line ult. for rhuburb read rhubarb.
Page 337, line 23, dele other.
Page 350, Motto, for phoenomena read phænomena.
Page 378, line 1, for on read independent of.

ESSAYS

MEDICAL

AND

EXPERIMENTAL.

VOL. II.

ESSAYS

MEDICAL AND EXPERIMENTAL,

ON THE

Following SUBJECTS;

1. On the COLUMBO ROOT.
2. On the ORCHIS ROOT.
3. On the WATERS of BUXTON and MATLOCK in Derbyshire.
4. On the Medicinal Uses of FIXED AIR.
5. On the antiseptic and sweetening powers, and on the varieties of FACTITIOUS AIR.
6. On the Noxious Vapours of CHARCOAL.
7. On the ATRABILIS.
8. On SEA SALT.
9. On COFFEE.

TO WHICH ARE ADDED,

SELECT HISTORIES OF DISEASES,

WITH REMARKS; AND

PROPOSALS FOR ESTABLISHING MORE ACCURATE AND COMPREHENSIVE BILLS OF MORTALITY.

BY

THOMAS PERCIVAL, M.D. F.R.S. & S.A.

——— *Sicut formica,*
Ore trahit quodcunque potest atque addit acervo.

HOR. Lib. I. Sat. I.

LONDON:

Printed for JOSEPH JOHNSON, No. 72, St. Paul's Church-Yard.

MDCCLXXIII.

THE

FOLLOWING

ESSAYS

ARE INSCRIBED

TO

THE RIGHT HONOURABLE

GEORGE

EARL OF STAMFORD,

&c. &c. &c.

AS A TRIBUTE

OF

ESTEEM, RESPECT, AND GRATITUDE,

BY

HIS LORDSHIP'S

MOST OBLIGED

AND MOST OBEDIENT SERVANT,

THOMAS PERCIVAL.

THE

PREFACE.

THE great Lord Verulam recommends the collecting of facts, obſervations, and experiments, as the beſt method of promoting the improvement of phyſic; and experience hath fully evinced the utility of ſuch a plan. In this way I am ambitious of contributing my mite to the general ſtock of medical knowledge; and ſhall think myſelf happy, if I can thus render the purſuit of my own inſtruction and amuſement, ſubſervient to the intereſts of my profeſſion, and to the general good of mankind.

THE Obſervations on the COLUMBO ROOT have been read at the College of Phyſicians, and before the Royal Society; and have been communicated to a conſiderable number of my friends and correſpondents, to ſome of whom this remedy was unknown, and by others applied only to the cure of the *cholera morbus*. During the courſe of the

the laſt year, I have had the ſatisfaction of receiving from them the ſtrongeſt teſtimonies of its efficacy, in a variety of diſorders. What I have advanced, therefore, in its favour, may be regarded, not as the concluſions of an individual, partial to a favourite remedy, but as facts ſupported by the experience of many learned and ingenious Phyſicians.

The diſſertation on the Orchis root has been honoured, by Doctor Hunter of York, with a place in the Georgical Eſſays, a uſeful and entertaining work on the ſubject of agriculture. But as it contains ſome experiments and obſervations on the medicinal quali-

ties

ties, as well as on the culture and preparation of this root, it is here reprinted, with a few corrections and additions.

THE papers on FACTITIOUS AIR form a part of an experimental inquiry into this interesting and curious branch of physics; in which the friendship, and too favourable opinion of Dr. Prieſtley firſt engaged me, in concert with himſelf. But this learned philoſopher, who poſſeſſes a happier genius, more leiſure, and better health than I am bleſt with, has carried his reſearches far beyond the limits of mine; and his pleaſing and wonderful diſcoveries in theſe almoſt trackleſs paths of ſcience, will reflect

flect the highest honour on his industry and abilities.

To this second volume of Experimental Essays, I have annexed a few select HISTORIES of DISEASES, agreeable to the plan of Lord Bacon, who advises Physicians "to revive the Hippocratic method of composing narratives of particular cases, in which the nature of the disease, the manner of treating it, and the consequences are to be specified; to attempt the cure of those diseases, which have been too boldly pronounced incurable; and to extend their inquiries into the powers of particular medicines, in the cure of particular disorders."(a)

THE

(a) De Augment. scient. l. iv. cap. 2.

The Proposals for eſtabliſhing more accurate and comprehenſive Bills of Mortality, were ſuggeſted by the peruſal of a Treatiſe on Reverſionary Payments, lately publiſhed by my friend Dr. Price; who employs his great mathematical knowledge, not in idle ſpeculation, or in the ſolution of amuſing problems, but in diſquiſitions at once curious, inſtructive, and of the higheſt importance to the intereſts of mankind. The Plan has been honoured with his approbation, and is likely to be carried into immediate execution at Mancheſter.

I cannot take my leave of the candid reader without intimating

ing, that though the experiments contained in theſe ſheets were made with great care, and are related with the ſtricteſt fidelity, I am ſenſible many inaccuracies may have eſcaped me; which thoſe will moſt readily excuſe, who have experienced the difficulties incident to ſuch reſearches. The Philoſopher has frequent occaſion to lament both the fallacy of his ſenſes, and the limited powers of his underſtanding. "You will wonder, ſays Mr. Boyle, in the preface to his philoſophical Eſſays, that I ſhould uſe ſo often *perhaps*, *it ſeems*, *'tis not improbable*, words which argue a diffidence of the truth of the opinions I incline to. But I have hitherto not unfrequently

quently found that what pleaſed me for a while, was ſoon after diſgraced by ſome further, or new experiment." Such is the imperfection of human knowledge, even when derived from evidence, which is uſually regarded as the moſt clear, and inconteſtible. And ſo true is the ſentiment of the comic poet,

Nunquam quiſquam ita bene ſubducta ratione ad vitam fuit,
Quin res, ætas, uſus aliquid apportet novi,
Aliquid admoneat, ut illa quæ te ſcire credas, neſcias,
Et quæ tibi putaris prima in experiundo repudies.

TERENT.

MANCHESTER,
1ſt Jan. 1773.

THE

CONTENTS.

Select

EXPE-

EXPERIMENTS

AND

OBSERVATIONS

ON THE

COLUMBO-ROOT.

——— *Symbolum aliquid, utcunque exiguum, in commune medicinæ ærarium contribuerem.*

SYDENHAM.

OBSERVATIONS AND EXPERIMENTS

ON THE

COLUMBO-ROOT.

THE Columbo-root, though a medicine of considerable efficacy, is not so generally known in practice as it deserves to be. Books, so far as my reading extends, are silent about it; and I have not hitherto been able to obtain any satisfactory information concerning its Natural History. The celebrated Linnæus is unacquainted with it. Dr. Watson made particular enquiry concerning it of an East-India Governor, and also of Mr. Loten, who was several years Governor of Ceylon. These Gentlemen

inform-

informed him only that the root was brought to Ceylon, and to our ſettlements, where it is called in the Portugueſe language *Raijs de Moſambique*. Doctor Hope, Profeſſor of Botany at Edinburgh, has tranſmitted to me the following account, which he received from Dr. Rainey, a Phyſician who reſided a long time in the Eaſt-Indies. The Columbo-root grew originally on the continent of Aſia, and was from thence tranſplanted to Columbo, a town in Ceylon, which now gives name to it, and ſupplies all India with it. The inhabitants of theſe countries have for a long time uſed it in diſorders of the ſtomach and bowels. They carry it about with them, and take it ſliced or ſcraped, in Madeira wine.

The Columbo-root comes to us in circular pieces, which are from half an inch to three inches in diameter; and divided into *fruſta*, which meaſure in length from two inches to one quarter of an inch.

inch. The ſides are covered with a thick, corrugated bark, of a dark brown hue on its external coat, but internally of a light yellow colour. The ſurfaces of the tranſverſe sections appear very unequal, higheſt at the edges, and forming a concavity towards the centre. On ſeparating this ſurface, the root is evidently ſeen to conſiſt of three *lamina*, viz. the cortical, which in the larger roots is a quarter of an inch thick; the ligneous, about half an inch; and the medullary which forms the center, and is near an inch in diameter. This laſt is much ſofter than the other parts, and when chewed ſeems very mucilaginous: A number of ſmall fibres run longitudinally through it, and appear on the ſurface. The cortical and ligneous parts are divided by a circular black line. All the thicker pieces have ſmall holes drilled through them, for the convenience of drying.

THIS root has an aromatic ſmell, but

is disagreeably bitter and slightly pungent to the taste, somewhat resembling mustard-seed, when it has lost by long keeping part of its essential oil. Yet though ungrateful to the taste, when received into the stomach it appears to be corroborant, antiseptic, sedative, and powerfully antiemetic.

IN the CHOLERA MORBUS it alleviates the violent *tormina*, checks the purging and vomiting, corrects the putrid tendency of the bile, quiets the inordinate motions of the bowels, and speedily recruits the exhausted strength of the patient. Mr. Johnson of Chester, a surgeon of eminence, who served ten years on board one of his Majesty's ships in the East Indies, and in 1756 had the care of an hospital-ship, gave the Columbo-root in that climate to a great number of patients, often twenty in a day, attacked with this disease. He seldom employed any means to promote the discharge of bile, or to cleanse

cleanſe the ſtomach and bowels, previous to its exhibition: And he generally found that it ſoon ſtopped the vomiting, which was the moſt fatal ſymptom, and that the purging and remaining complaints, quickly yielded to the ſame remedy. The mortality on board his ſhip, after he uſed this medicine, was remarkably leſs than in the other ſhips of the ſame fleet; and this difference he attributes entirely to the good effects of the Columbo-root in this fatal diſorder. The doſe he gave was from half a drachm to two drachms of the powder, every three or four hours, more or leſs according to the urgency of the ſymptoms.

THOUGH Columbo-root does not ſeem to poſſeſs much, if any degree of aſtringency, yet I have often obſerved very ſalutary effects from its uſe, in DIARRHOEAS, and even in the DYSENTERY. In the firſt ſtage of theſe diſorders, when aſtringents would be hurtful, this root may be prescribed with safety and advantage, for by its antispasmodic powers, it corrects the irregular action of the *primæ viæ*. But as a cordial, tonic, and antiseptic remedy, it answers better when given towards their decline.

I HAVE more than once experienced its efficacy in the vomitings which attend the BILIOUS CHOLIC; and in such cases where an emetic is thought necessary, after administering a small dose of ipecacuan, the stomach may be washed with an infusion of Columbo-root. This will answer the purposes of an evacuant, as well as chamomile tea, and will tend to prevent those violent and convulsive reachings which in irritable habits, abounding with bile, are sometimes excited by the mildest emetic. The efficacy of ipecacuan in the cholic, given in small doses, is well known; and perhaps its operation as an antispasmodic may in some measure depend on the nausea which it produces.

But

But unfortunately it often occaſions very ſevere ſickneſs and vomiting, and thus aggravates the diſorder, by inducing a new and moſt diſtreſſing ſymptom. Perhaps (for I ſpeak not from experience) if it were combined with ſome grateful aromatic, and adminiſtered in an infuſion of Columbo, prepared with mint water, this troubleſome effect might be obviated.

In bilious fevers, fifteen or twenty grains of this root, with an equal or double quantity of vitriolated tartar, given every four, five, or ſix hours, produce very beneficial effects. The neutral ſalt abates the febrile heat, allays thirſt, and brings on a gentle ſalutary *diarrhœa*; whilſt the Columbo-root ſupports the ſtrength of the patient, obviates the nauſea and ſickneſs to which he is ſo much diſpoſed, and powerfully checks the ſeptic ferment in the *primæ viæ*. When the belly is ſufficiently ſoluble, an infuſion of it may be directed, well acidulated

lated with *elixir vitriol. dulc.** Is it not probable, that the Columbo may be highly serviceable in the malignant, YELLOW FEVER of the West-Indies? This fever is always attended with great sickness, violent reachings, and a copious discharge of bile. The vomiting recurs at

* DR. HAYGARTH, a very ingenious Physician at Chester, has lately by my recommendation, made trial of the Columbo-root, in a fever of the bilious kind, which has been epidemic at Namptwich, and in other parts of Cheshire; and he has favoured me with the following account of his success. "After the *primæ viæ* have been sufficiently unloaded of their bilious, and other putrescent contents, I find the Columbo-root a most useful remedy, in allaying the nausea and reachings, to which the patients are liable. In this fever, though the remissions are very evident, and the accessions generally marked with chills and other symptoms of an intermittent, yet the bark appears to do more harm than good, as it occasions an increase of feverish heat, and a parched tongue. The Columbo in these cases seems to supply its place most admirably, by correcting the bile, restoring the proper tone of the stomach, and of the whole habit. It also prevents relapses, to which in this fever, the patients are particularly disposed."

"SUCH

at ſhort intervals, often becomes almoſt inceſſant, and an incredible quantity of bile is ſometimes evacuated, in a few hours.

CHILDREN during DENTITION, are frequently ſubject to ſevere vomitings and diarrhœas. In theſe caſes the Columbo-root is an uſeful remedy; and I have ſeen almoſt inſtant relief procured by it, when other efficacious medicines had been tried in vain. The more effectually to correct the acidities which at ſuch times uſually prevail, a little chalk or magneſia may be combined with it.

THE

"SUCH have been the good effects of the Columbo-root in the caſes which have fallen under my own obſervation; but a judicious Apothecary informs me, that he has often ſeen it fail of ſucceſs in this fever, which in no reſpect ſeems wonderful. It is not ſuppoſed that Columbo has any febrifuge quality, ſimilar to antimony, or Peruvian bark. By correcting the putrid bile it deſtroys the *fomes* which aggravates the fever, and produces many of its moſt dangerous ſymptoms. When bilious fevers are epidemical, does it not ſeem a probable remedy to prevent the diſeaſe?"

THE Columbo-root is extremely beneficial in a LANGUID STATE of the STOMACH, attended with want of appetite, indigeſtion, nauſea, and flatulence. It may be given either in ſubſtance, with ſome grateful aromatic, or infuſed in Madeira wine, and during the uſe of it, gentle doſes of the tincture of rhubarb, or of any other ſtrengthening and cordial purgative, ſhould occaſionally be preſcribed. If the bile appear to be defective, a ſufficient quantity of ox gall, carefully evaporated to the conſiſtence of an extract, may be mixed with the powder of Columbo, and the maſs reduced into pills. In this manner I have frequently taken the Columbo-root myſelf, and have generally found my appetite increaſed, and my digeſtion improved by it.

HABITUAL VOMITING, when it proceeds from a weakneſs or irritability of the ſtomach, from an irregular gout, from acidities,

acidities, from acrimonious bile, or an increaſed and depraved ſecretion of the pancreatic juice, are greatly relieved by the uſe of Columbo-root, in conjunction with aromatics, chalybeates, or the teſtaceous powders. But this diſeaſe often ariſes, when ſuch a cauſe is leaſt ſuſpected, from an affection of the kidneys. Under ſuch circumſtances, demulcents, and gentle diuretics, are the moſt ſucceſsful remedies; though I have frequently obſerved temporary relief procured by a light infuſion of this root in mint water.

SUCH an infuſion ſucceeds better than any other medicine I have tried, in the nauſea and vomiting occaſioned by PREGNANCY. But it is ſometimes neceſſary to premiſe venæſection, and always expedient to keep the patient's body moderately open with magneſia.

I COULD

I COULD illuſtrate the truth of theſe obſervations, by a variety of caſes; but to enter into ſo minute a detail would be equally unneceſſary and uninteresting. I ſhall confine myſelf therefore to the relation of a few hiſtories, which exemplify the peculiar, or if the expreſſion be allowable, ſpecific qualities of the Columbo-root.

CASE I.

T. H. of Newton-lane near Mancheſter, in the month of Auguſt 1770, from expoſure to cold when overheated with hard labour, was attacked with a ſevere purging and vomiting, accompanied with violent pain in his ſtomach and bowels. He continued in this miſerable condition twenty-four hours before I ſaw him, and his ſtrength was then nearly exhauſted. I directed two ſcruples of the powder of Columbo-

Columbo-root, to be given every three or four hours in pepper-mint water. This remedy afforded almoſt immediate relief; but the patient returning too ſoon to his occupation, had a relapſe, and was again reſtored to health by the ſame medicine.

*CASE II.

W. W. Auguſt 31. 1770, had been ſeized with a looſeneſs three days before, which had gradually increaſed, and for the laſt four hours, been moſt violent, attended with frequent vomiting, and cramps in his extremities. He was directed to take a ſcruple of the powder of Columbo every two hours, and had neither vomiting, nor purging after the firſt doſe. Nine doſes reſtored him to perfect health.

* Communicated by Dr Haygarth.

CASE

*CASE III.

April, 1771. Mrs. P—— about the beginning of the third week of her confinement in child-bed, began to complain of great pain, fullneſs, and uneaſineſs in the bowels, accompanied with frequent and copious evacuations by ſtool. What was diſcharged had the colour and conſiſtence of cream. The pulſe was from 100 to 115. The tongue had a whitiſh fur; and the ſkin was often dry and hot. The evacuations by ſtool, and the other ſymptoms were always much more conſiderable during the night, than in the day. Ipecacuanha as an emetic, opiates, elixir of vitriol, and other cooling reſtringents, afforded no relief. A ſtrong infuſion of the Columbo-root in cinnamon tea, was then given with the deſired effect. After every tea-cup full of the infuſion

* Communicated by Dr. Dobſon of Liverpool.

fuſion the patient found herſelf better; the painful ſenſations were relieved, and the evacuations diminiſhed. In about five days ſhe was entirely cured.

CASE IV.

R. N. Eſq. aged 26, the latter end of June 1771, when the weather was extremely hot, was ſeized with the uſual ſymptoms of a fever. An emetic and gentle cathartic were adminiſtered, and ſaline draughts were directed to be taken at proper intervals. He perſiſted in this courſe two or three days, without any ſenſible relief. A continual nauſea, and frequent vomitings of green bile now came on. The ſkin was hot and dry; the pulſe beat an hundred and twenty ſtrokes in a minute; the tongue was foul; the belly not ſufficiently ſoluble, notwithſtanding the free uſe of ſtrawberries, and other fruit was enjoined; and he complained of great pain in his head and back, attended with univerſal laſſitude. A clyſter was immediately injected; and two ſcruples of vitriolated tartar were given every four hours, in three ſpoonful of the infuſion of Columbo. The firſt doſe almoſt inſtantly alleviated the nauſea and ſickneſs, and the continuance of the ſame remedy entirely prevented their return; whilſt the gentle diarrhœa produced by the neutral ſalt, mitigated all the febrile ſymptoms. On the eleventh day he had two bloody ſtools, and as his conſtitution was feeble and relaxed, the Peruvian bark combined with aſtringents was adminiſtered without delay: The hæmorrhage was ſoon checked, and the patient gradually recovered his uſual health and ſtrength.

CASE V.

JUNE 2d, 1771. Mr. W.'s ſon, aged 2, with other ſymptoms of dentition, had ſevere

ſevere purging and vomiting, which continuing three days, reduced him to the loweſt degree of weakneſs. I directed five grains of Columbo-root, and three grains of *pulv. e chel. c. c.* to be taken every two hours. The vomiting was ſtopped by the firſt doſe; the looſeneſs was ſoon after checked, and in two days the child recovered his uſual ſtrength.

I SHALL now proceed to relate the experiments which I have made on the Columbo-root.

EXPERIMENT I.

TWO drachms of Columbo-root powdered, were infuſed without heat, in four ounces of each of the following *menſtrua*. 1. Rectified ſpirit of wine. 2. French brandy. 3. Madeira wine. 4. White wine. 5. Diſtilled water. 6. White wine vinegar. 7. Hard ſpring water. After twenty-four hours digeſtion, the tinctures, &c. were filtered through paper, and equal quantities of each, and of their reſpective *menſtrua* were weighed with great exactneſs, and compared together. The tincture made with rectified ſpirit of wine, appeared by its taſte, colour, and ſuperiour ſpecific gravity to the ſimple ſpirit, to be conſiderably ſtronger than the reſt; whoſe degree of impregnation, ſeemed by theſe teſts, to be exactly in the order in which I have enumerated the ſeveral *menſtrua* employed in their preparation. It ſhould be remarked, that the watery infuſion of Columbo-root is more periſhable than that of other bitters. In twenty-four hours a copious precipitation takes place in it, and in two days it becomes ropy and even muſty.

EXPERIMENT II.

THE addition of orange peel renders the infuſion of Columbo-root leſs ungrateful

grateful to the palate. An ounce of the powdered root, half an ounce of orange-peel, two ounces of French brandy, and fourteen ounces of water, macerated twelve hours without heat, and then filtered through paper, afforded a ſufficiently ſtrong, and tolerably pleaſant infuſion.

EXPERIMENT III.

TWELVE ounces of Columbo-root in groſs powder were digeſted four days in three pints of rectified ſpirit of wine. The tincture was then filtered; and the *reſiduum* boiled repeatedly in a ſufficient quantity of water, till it yielded no taſte to the liquor. The decoctions, having been carefully percolated, were evaporated over a gentle fire in the common method, till about three quarts only remained. The evaporation was then continued in the vapour bath, and when nearly finiſhed, the tincture, from which a part of the ſpirit had been previouſly drawn by the alembic, was gradually added, and the whole reduced to a pilular conſiſtence, retaining the entire flavour of the Columbo, free from the leaſt degre of *empyreuma*, and weighing eight ounces and two drachms. The ſpirit diſtilled from the tincture was neither impregnated with the taſte nor odour of the root; which is a proof that no volatile parts were diſſipated by this proceſs. This experiment was made at my requeſt, by Mr. Henry, an ingenious and accurate Apothecary in Mancheſter. I have frequently uſed the extract of Columbo, and find it equal, if not ſuperior in efficacy to the powder.

EXPERIMENT IV.

EQUAL weights, viz. about two drachms of beef, cut into ſmall pieces, were macerated ſeparately in an ounce of a cold infuſion of the Peruvian bark, and of Columbolumbo-root, filtered and prepared in a manner exactly ſimilar. The experiment was made in the month of July, the weather was uncommonly warm, and the bottles were placed in a window which had a ſouthern aſpect. In forty-eight hours the beef in the infuſion of Columbo-root had acquired a ſlightly putrid fœtor, whilſt that in the infuſion of bark remained perſectly ſweet, and continued ſo ten hours longer. Two drachms of beef macerated in cold water, and intended for a ſtandard, became putrid in twenty-four hours, under the circumſtances above deſcribed.

EXPERIMENT V.

THE putrid beef employed as a ſtandard in the laſt experiment, was divided into two equal parts, to one of which was added an ounce of the infuſion of Columbo-root; to the other the ſame quantity of the infuſion of Peruvian bark. After ſix hours maceration, the pieces of fleſh had loſt much of their putrid fœtor; but that in the infuſion of Columbo-root, was more offenſive than the other.

EXPERIMENT VI.

To ſeveral phials, each containing three drachms of putrid ox gall, and two drachms of ſaliva, were added equal quantities, viz. an ounce of, 1. the infuſion of Columbo-root; 2. the infuſion of Peruvian bark; 3. the infuſion of chamomile flowers; 4. ſpring water: the laſt was intended as a ſtandard. The phials were placed in a water bath, heated to about 100 degrees of Farenheit's thermometer. When the infuſion of bark was mixed with the putrid gall and ſaliva, it inſtantly produced a coagulation of the gall, and conſiderably increaſed the fœtor of it. Whereas the infuſion of Columbo united perfectly with it, it, and very powerfully corrected its offensive ſmell. The infuſion of chamomile occaſioned no change in the bile, either with reſpect to its fœtor or fluidity. After three hours digeſtion, the putrid ſmell of the gall was much abated, in all the phials but the ſtandard, and even in that was leſs perceptible than at firſt. In ſix hours no fœtor could be perceived, except in the ſtandard; and the mixture with the bark had acquired a vinous ſmell, and emitted many air bubbles. In twelve hours the odour of the gall was ſenſible, but not offenſive in the mixtures with Columbo and chamomile: The bark now fermented leſs, and had loſt ſomewhat of its vinous ſmell. In twenty-four hours the ſtandard became extremely putrid; the mixture with bark was ſour; the Columbo and chamomile were ſtill ſweet; but in thirty hours they became putrid, and in forty hours they were highly offenſive.

THE

The instantaneous effect of the infusion of Columbo in correcting the putridity of the ox gall, serves in some measure to explain its action in the *cholera morbus*, and other diseases, attended with a redundance and depravation of the bile: And at the same time it obviates all objection to the use of this remedy, previous to any artificial evacuations, in the first stage of such disorders; a practice which indeed is justified by its success. The coagulation and increased fœtor of the gall, which the infusion of bark occasioned, very well account for the disagreement of that medicine with the stomach in the yellow fever of the West-Indies. Doctor Hillary laments that though strongly indicated, it cannot be retained, even under the pleasantest form. Is it not probable that the Columbo-root, which so readily unites with, and so quickly sweetens putrid bile, would prove very salutary in this dangerous and malignant disease?

EXPE-

EXPERIMENT VII.

Equal quantities, viz. an ounce of water, of the infuſions of Columbo-root, Peruvian bark, and chamomile flowers, were added to four phials, each containing three drachms of freſh ox gall, and two drachms of ſaliva. The bottles were then placed at ſuch a diſtance from the fire, as to be kept blood-warm. In ſix hours all the mixtures except the ſtandard, were in fermentation. The infuſion of bark emitted moſt, and that of Columbo the feweſt air bubbles: The former alſo had acquired a vinous ſmell. In twenty-four hours the ſtandard became putrid. In forty-eight hours the infuſion of bark was ſour, that of chamomile ſlightly putrid; but that of Columbo-root was perfectly ſweet, and continued ſo many hours afterwards, when the phials were ſet aſide.

N. B. The infuſion of bark when mixed

mixed with the recent gall produced a coagulation, but not in ſo great a degree as when combined with putrid bile.

Sir John Pringle found that chamomile flowers reſiſt the purefaction of animal fleſh, more powerfully than Jeſuit's bark; and from one of the preceding experiments it appears that in this reſpect, bark is more antiſeptic than Columbo-root. But as a preſervative of the *bile* from putridity, this root ſurpaſſes *chamomile flowers*, without producing like the bark any changes in it by fermentation. Hence may be juſtly inferred the utility of Columbo-root in diſorders of a putrid tendency, and in an impaired digeſtion from corrupted bile, or vitiated and unſound ſaliva.

EXPERIMENT VIII.

To determine the comparative action of Columbo-root, on the fermentation of of food in the ſtomach; I digeſted in the water bath three alimentary mixtures, prepared of two drachms of the crumb of bread, the ſame quantity of roaſted mutton chopped very ſmall, and an ounce of the infuſions of Columbo-root, chamomile flowers, and muſtard ſeed. The ingredients of each mixture were well united by triture in a mortar; and a fourth phial was provided as a ſtandard, which contained the proportions beforementioned of bread and mutton, with half an ounce of water, and the ſame quantity of ſaliva. In twelve hours the ſtandard began to ferment; in thirty hours an inteſtine motion was perceptible in the other mixtures, but appeared to be leaſt in the phial which contained the Columbo-root. In forty-eight hours the ſtandard became ſour. The third day the mixture with the infuſion of chamomile was alſo ſour. The two remaining phials, viz. the infuſions of Columbo and of muſtard, were now placed by the fire,

where

where they continued ten days, without ſhewing the leaſt ſigns either of acidity, or of putrefaction.

The reſemblance between the taſte of muſtard and of Columbo-root, induced me to try their comparative action on alimentary fermentation. And it appears that they concur in moderating, without ſuſpending the proceſs of digeſtion. This property gives Columbo-root the advantage over other bitters, in ſuch diſorders of the ſtomach, as are attended with a violent fermentation of the food, with flatulence, and great acidity. And if a ſtimulus be wanting to excite this organ to a quicker expulſion of its contents, ſome grateful aromatic may be combined with it: Or perhaps muſtard-ſeed would equally anſwer this intention, without increaſing, like the ſpices, the generation of air. This experiment proves the remarkable efficacy of the Columbo in preventing acidities; and the ſucceeding one no leſs clearly

clearly evinces its power of neutralizing them.

EXPERIMENT IX.

To an ounce of the infusions of chamomile flowers, of Columbo-root, and of Peruvian bark, were added twenty drops of vinegar. The infusion of Columbo entirely neutralized the acid, that of chamomile flowers in some measure covered the taste of it; but the infusion of bark was evidently sour both to the taste and smell, and it required twenty drops more of vinegar, to render the infusion of Columbo equally acidulated with that of the bark.

EXPERIMENT X.

To ascertain the action of Columbo-root on the heart and arteries, I took a scruple

ſcruple of the powder in a ſmall glaſs of ſpring water, at ſeven o'clock in the evening. My ſtomach was empty; I had been ſitting at reſt an hour; and my pulſe then beat ſeventy-four ſtrokes in a minute. I continued to ſit ſtill half an hour longer, and every fifth minute examined my pulſe, but could perceive no variation, either in its regularity, fullneſs, or velocity. The ſucceeding evening I repeated the ſame experiment, with the precautions I had before obſerved, and increaſed the doſe of Columbo to half a drachm. At the time I ſwallowed the powder, my pulſe beat eighty ſtrokes in a minute; in ten minutes it became fuller, and ſlower by three ſtrokes, and continued to beat the ſame number, viz. ſeventy-ſeven for three quarters of an hour.

THIS experiment ſhews that the Columbo-root does not belong to the claſs of heating bitters: It may therefore be uſed with propriety and advantage in the

pthiſis

pthiſis pulmonalis, and in hectical caſes, to correct acrimony, and ſtrengthen the organs of digeſtion. The Peruvian bark often proves oppreſſive to the ſtomach in ſuch diſorders, and ſometimes excites a *diarrhœa*. But the Columbo-root occaſions no diſturbance, and agrees very well with a milk diet, as it abates flatulence, and is indiſpoſed to acidity.

ON THE PREPARATION, CULTURE, AND USE OF THE ORCHIS ROOT.

Fungar vice cotis.

HOR.

ON THE

PREPARATION, CULTURE, AND USE

OF THE

ORCHIS ROOT.

SALEP is a preparation of the root of Orchis, or Dogſtones, of which many ſpecies are enumerated by Botanical writers. The *Orchis maſcula, Linn. ſp. pl.* is the moſt valued, although the roots of ſome of the palmated ſorts, particularly of the *Orchis latifolia*, are found to anſwer almoſt equally well. This plant flouriſhes in various parts of Europe and Aſia, and grows in our country ſpontaneouſly, and in great abundance. It is aſſiduouſly cultivated in the Eaſt, and the root of it forms a conſiderable part of the diet of the inhabitants of Turkey, Perſia, and Syria. A dry and not very fertile ſoil is beſt adapted to its growth. An ingenious friend of mine, in order to collect the ſeed, tranſplanted a number of the Orchiſes into a meadow, where he had prepared a bed well manured for their reception. The next ſpring few of them appeared, and not one came to maturity, their roots being black and half rotten. The ſame gentleman informed me, that he had never been able to raiſe any plant from the ſeed of the wild Orchis; but he aſcribes his want of ſucceſs to the wetneſs of the ſituation in which he reſides. I have now before me a ſeed pod of the Orchis, the contents of which to the naked eye, ſeem to be ſeed corrupted and turned to duſt, but when viewed through a microſcope appear evidently to be organized, and would I doubt not with proper culture germinate, and produce a thriving crop of plants. The propereſt time for gathering the roots is when the ſeed

ſeed is formed, and the ſtalk is ready to fall, becauſe the new bulb, of which the ſalep is made, is then arrived to its full maturity, and may be diſtinguiſhed from the old one, by a white bud riſing from the top of it, which is the germ of the Orchis of the ſucceeding year.

SEVERAL methods of preparing ſalep have been propoſed and practiſed. Geoffroy has delivered a very judicious proceſs for this purpoſe, in the *Hiſtoire de l'Academie Royale des Sciences* 1740; and Retzius, in the Swediſh Tranſactions 1764, has improved Geoffroy's method. But Mr. Moult of Rochdale has lately favoured the public with a new manner of curing the Orchis root, and as I have ſeen many ſpecimens of his ſalep, at leaſt equal if not ſuperior to any brought from the Levant, I can recommend the following, which is his proceſs, from my own knowledge of its ſucceſs.

The new root is to be waſhed in water, and the fine brown ſkin which covers it is to be ſeparated by means of a ſmall bruſh, or by dipping the root in hot water, and rubbing it with a coarſe linen cloth. When a ſufficient number of roots have been thus cleaned, they are to be ſpread on a tin plate, and placed in an oven heated to the uſual degree, where they are to remain ſix or ten minutes, in which time they will have loſt their milky whiteneſs, and acquired a tranſparency like horn, without any diminution of bulk. Being arrived at this ſtate they are to be removed, in order to dry and harden in the air, which will require ſeveral days to effect; or by uſing a very gentle heat, they may be finiſhed in a few hours. *(a)*

Salep thus prepared, may be afforded in this part of England, where labour bears

(a) Vid. a Letter from Mr. John Moult to the Author, containing a new method of preparing Salep.
Phil. Tranſact. Vol. 59.

bears a high value, at about eight pence or ten pence per pound. And it might be ſold ſtill cheaper, if the Orchis were to be cured, without ſeparating from it the brown ſkin which covers it: A troubleſome part of the proceſs, and which does not contribute to render the root, either more palatable or ſalutary. Whereas the foreign ſalep is now ſold at five or ſix ſhillings per pound.

The culture of the Orchis therefore is an object highly deſerving of encouragement, from all the lovers of agriculture. And as the root, if introduced into common uſe, would furniſh a cheap, wholeſome, and moſt nutritious article of diet, the growth of it would be ſufficiently profitable to the farmer.

Salep is ſaid to contain the greateſt quantity of vegetable nouriſhment in the ſmalleſt bulk. Hence a very judicious writer, to prevent the dreadful calamity of of famine at ſea, has lately propoſed that the powder of it ſhould conſtitute part of the proviſions of every ſhip's company. This powder and portable ſoup, diſſolved in boiling water, form a rich thick jelly, capable of ſupporting life for a conſiderable length of time. An ounce of each of theſe articles, with two quarts of boiling water, will be ſufficient ſubſiſtence for a man a day *(b)*; and as being a mixture of animal, and vegetable food, muſt prove more nouriſhing than double the quantity of rice cake, made by boiling rice in water; this laſt however ſailors are often obliged ſolely to ſubſiſt upon for ſeveral months, eſpecially in voyages to Guinea, when the bread and flour are exhauſted, and the beef and pork, having been ſalted in

(b) Portable ſoup is ſold at half a crown per pound; ſalep, if cultivated in our own country, might be afforded at ten pence per pound; the day's ſubſiſtence would therefore amount only to two pence halfpenny.

in hot countries, are become unfit for uſe.*

But as a wholeſome nouriſhment, rice is much inferior to ſalep. I digeſted ſeveral alimentary mixtures prepared of mutton and water, beat up with bread, ſea biſcuit, ſalep, rice flour, ſago powder, potato, old cheeſe, &c. in a heat equal to that of the human body. In forty-eight hours they had all acquired a vinous ſmell, and were in briſk fermentation, except the mixture with rice, which did not emit many air bubbles, and was but little changed. The third day ſeveral of the mixtures were ſweet, and continued to ferment; others had loſt their inteſtine motion, and were ſour; but the one which contained the rice was become putrid. From this experiment it appears that rice as an aliment, is ſlow of fermentation,

* Vid. Dr. Lind's Appendix to his Eſſay on the Diſeaſes of Hot Climates.

mentation, and a very weak corrector of putrefaction. It is therefore an improper diet for hospital patients; but more particularly for sailors, in long voyages, because it is incapable of preventing, and will not contribute much to check the progress of that fatal disease, the sea scurvy. (c) Under certain circumstances rice seems disposed of itself, without mixture, to become putrid. For by long keeping it sometimes acquires an offensive fœtor. Nor can it be considered as a very nutritive kind of food, on account of its difficult solubility in the stomach. Experience confirms the truth of this conclusion;

(c) CHEESE is now become a considerable article of ship provisions. When mellowed by age it ferments readily with flesh and water, but separates a rancid oil, which seems incapable of any further change, and must, as a septic, be pernicious in the scurvy. For rancidity appears to be a species of putrefaction. The same objection may be urged, with still greater propriety, against the use of cheese in hospitals; because convalescents are so liable to relapses, that the slightest error of diet may occasion them. Vid. Percival's Letter to Mr. Aikin, Thoughts on Hospitals, p. 95.

on; for it is obſerved by the planters in the Weſt-Indies, that the negroes grow thin, and are leſs able to work, whilſt they ſubſiſt upon rice.

Salep has the ſingular property of concealing the taſte of ſalt water *(d)*; a circumſtance of the higheſt importance at ſea, when there is a ſcarcity of freſh water. I diſſolved a drachm and a half of common ſalt in a pint of the mucilage of ſalep, ſo liquid as to be potable, and the ſame quantity in a pint of ſpring water. The ſalep was by no means diſagreeable to the taſte, but the water was rendered extremely unpalatable.

This experiment ſuggeſted to me the trial of the Orchis root as a corrector of acidity, a property which would render it a very uſeful diet for children. But the ſolution of it, when mixed with vinegar,

(d) Vid. Dr. Lind's Appendix.

negar, ſeemed only to dilute, like an equal proportion of water, and not to cover its ſharpneſs.

Salep however appears by my experiments, to retard the acetous fermentation of milk, and conſequently would be a good lithing for milk pottage, eſpecially in large towns, where the cattle being fed upon ſour draft, muſt yield aceſcent milk.

Salep in a certain proportion, which I have not yet been able to aſcertain, would be a very uſeful and profitable addition to bread. I directed one ounce of the powder to be diſſolved in a quart of water, and the mucilage to be be mixed with a ſufficient quantity of flour, ſalt, and yeaſt. The flour amounted to two pounds, the yeaſt to two ounces, and the ſalt to eighty grains. The loaf when baked was remarkably well fermented, and weighed three pounds two ounces.

Another

Another loaf, made with the ſame quantity of flour, &c. weighed two pounds and twelve ounces; from which it appears, that the ſalep, though uſed in ſo ſmall a proportion, increaſed the gravity of the loaf ſix ounces, by abſorbing and retaining more water than the flour alone was capable of. Half a pound of flour, and an ounce of ſalep were mixed together, and the water added according to the uſual method of preparing bread. The loaf when baked weighed thirteen ounces and a half; and would probably have been heavier, if the ſalep had been previouſly diſſolved in about a pint of water. But it ſhould be remarked, that the quantity of flour uſed in this trial was not ſufficient to conceal the peculiar taſte of the ſalep.

The reſtorative, mucilaginous, and demulcent qualities of the Orchis root render it of conſiderable uſe in various diſeaſes. In the ſea ſcurvy it powerfully obtunds

obtunds the acrimony of the fluids, and at the ſame time is eaſily aſſimulated into a mild and nutritious chyle. In diarrhœas and the dyſentery it is highly ſerviceable, by ſheathing the internal coat of the inteſtines, by abating irritation, and gently correcting putrefaction. In the ſymptomatic fever, which ariſes from the abſorption of pus, from ulcers in the lungs, from wounds, or from amputation, ſalep uſed plentifully is an admirable demulcent, and well adapted to reſiſt that diſſolution of the *craſis* of the blood, which is ſo evident in theſe caſes. And by the ſame mucilaginous quality, it is equally efficacious in the ſtrangury, and dyſury; eſpecially in the latter when ariſing from a venereal cauſe, becauſe the diſcharge of urine is then attended with the moſt exquiſite pain, from the ulcerations about the neck of the bladder, and through the courſe of the *urethra*. I have found it alſo an uſeful

ful aliment for patients who labour under the ſtone or gravel. (e)

From theſe obſervations, ſhort and imperfect as they are, I hope it will ſufficiently appear that the culture of the Orchis root is an object of conſiderable importance

(e) The ancient chemiſts ſeem to have entertained a very high opinion of the virtues of the Orchis root, of which the following quotation from the SECRETA SECRETORUM of Raymund Lully, affords a diverting proof. The work is dated 1565.

SEXTA HERBA,

Satirion.

"Satirion herba eſt pluribus nota, hujus radicis collecta ad pondus lib. 4. die 20 menſis Januarij, contunde fortiter & maſſam contuſam pone in ollam de aurichalcum habente in cooperculo 20 foramina minuta ſicut athomi, & pone intus cũ prædicta meſſa lactis vaccini calidi ſicut mulgetur de vacca ℔. 3. & mellis libram 1. vini aromatici ℔. 2. & repone per dies 20. ad ſolem & conſerua & utere."

"Iſtius itaq; doſis ad pondus 3. 4. & hora diei decima exhibita mulieri poſt ipſius menſtrua eadem nocte cõcipiet ſi vir cum ea agat."

importance to the public, and highly worthy of encouragement from all the patrons of agriculture. That taſte for experiment, which characteriſes the preſent age, and which has ſo amazingly enlarged the boundaries of ſcience, now animates the RATIONAL FARMER, who fears not to deviate from the beaten track, whenever improvements are ſuggeſted, or uſeful projects are pointed out to him. Much has been already done for the advancement of agriculture; but the earth ſtill teems with treaſures which remain to be explored. The bounties of nature are inexhauſtible, and will forever employ the art, and reward the induſtry of man.

MISCEL-

MISCELLANEOUS EXPERIMENTS AND OBSERVATIONS

—— *Alij hinc saltem, hac data via, felicioribus freti ingenijs, rei rectius gerendæ et melius inquirendi occasionem capiant.*

G. HARVEIJ. Op.

EXPERIMENTS AND OBSERVATIONS

ON THE WATERS OF

BUXTON AND MATLOCK,

In DERBYSHIRE.

THE water of St. Ann's well at BUXTON, is found, by analysis, to contain calcareous earth, fossil alkali, and sea salt; but in very small proportions. For a gallon of the water, when evaporated, yields only twenty-three or twenty-four grains of sediment. It strikes a slight green colour with syrup of violets, suffers no change from an infusion of galls, from the fixed vegetable alkali, or from the

 mineral

mineral acids; becomes milky with the volatile alkali, and with *ſaccharum ſaturni*; and lets fall a precipitate on the addition of a few drops of a ſolution of ſilver, in the nitrous acid. The ſpecific gravity of this water is preciſely equal to that of rain water, when their temperatures are the ſame; but it weighs four grains in a pint lighter, when firſt taken from the ſpring. The temperature of the bath is about 82 degrees of Farenheit's thermometer; that of St. Ann's well, as it is a ſmaller body of water, and expoſed to the open air, is ſomewhat leſs. The water is tranſparent, ſparkling, and highly grateful to the palate. *(a)*

In October 1769, I paſſed a few days at Buxton; and during my ſtay there amuſed myſelf with the following experiments

(a) I am indebted to the information of the judicious and worthy Phyſician, who attends at Buxton, for ſome of theſe facts.

ments on the effects of the water of St. Ann's well on my pulse.

EXPERIMENT I.

October 12th. EIGHT o'clock in the morning. The day cold and moist. My pulse beat 84 strokes in a minute. I drank at the well the third of a pint of water, and using every necessary precaution, examined my pulse at certain intervals of time. In five minutes pulse 80. In ten minutes pulse 80, fuller and harder. In twenty minutes pulse 85. In half an hour pulse 90.

EXPERIMENT II.

ELEVEN o'clock a. m. Two hours after breakfast. The air warm and serene. Pulse 90. I repeated the draught of water. In seven minutes pulse 109. In fifteen minutes pulse 103. In thirty minutes pulſe 100. Head ach. In an hour and a half pulſe 95. Head ach abated.

EXPERIMENT III.

October 13th. Eight o'clock in the morning. The day cold. Pulſe 92. I drank the quantity of water above-mentioned. In five minutes pulſe 86. In fifteen minutes pulſe 86, full and hard. In twenty minutes pulſe 100. In half an hour pulſe 92.

From the firſt and third experiments it appears that the coldneſs of the morning counteracted, for a time, the effects of the Buxton water, and reduced the vibrations of my pulſe from 84 to 80, and from 92 to 86. But the ſtimulus of the water ſoon became ſuperiour to the ſedative powers of the cold to which I was expoſed; for within the ſpace of half an hour my pulſe roſe to 90 in the firſt, and

to

to 100 ſtrokes in the ſecond trial. At eleven o'clock before noon, when the air was warm and ſerene, the water in a much ſhorter time exerted its full force, increaſing the velocity of my pulſe from 90 to 109 vibrations in a minute.

THESE experiments evince the heating quality of Buxton water, and ſuggeſt to us the precautions to be obſerved in the uſe of it. Small quantities only ſhould be drunk at once, and frequently repeated; the belly ſhould be kept ſoluble with lenitive electuary, or any other mild purgative; and at the beginning of the courſe, the patient may be directed to ſuffer the water to remain a few ſeconds in the glaſs, before he ſwallows it. For this celebrated ſpring abounds with a mineral ſpirit, or mephitic air, in which its ſtimulus, and indeed its efficacy reſides, and which is quickly diſſipated by expoſure to the air.

THE hon[ble]. and ingenious Mr. Cavendiſh has ſhewn, by his Experiments on Rathboneplace water, Philoſ. Tranſact. vol. 57, that calcareous earths may be rendered ſoluble in water, by furniſhing them with more than their natural proportion of fixed air. And it has lately been diſcovered that iron alſo may be ſuſpended by this principle, in the ſame *menſtruum*. (*b*) It appeared, therefore, highly probable to me, that a chalybeate impregnation might, with great facility, be communicated to the Buxton water, when freſh drawn from the ſpring; a quality which in many caſes would add greatly to its medicinal efficacy. I ſuggeſted the trial to Mr. Buxton, a worthy and ſenſible Apothecary near the wells, who has lately, at my requeſt, made the following experiment.

EXPE-

(*b*) Vid. Mr. Lane's Experiments, Phil. Tranſ. vol. 59.

EXPERIMENT IV.

A QUART bottle, containing two drachms of iron filings, was filled by immerſion, with the water of St. Ann's well, corked and agitated briſkly under the ſurface of the water. It was then ſuffered to remain in the well till the filings had ſubſided, when the water was carefully decanted into a half pint glaſs. To this were added three drops of the tincture of galls, which immediately occaſioned a deep purple colour; and the tranſparency was preſently reſtored, by a few drops of the acid of vitriol; evident proofs that a ſolution of the iron was effected in a few minutes. The water alſo, without the tincture of galls, had a chalybeate taſte, and left an agreeable aſtringency upon the palate.

BY this experiment it appears that a warm chalybeate, abounding with a mineral

neral ſpirit, and grateful to the taſte, may with very little trouble be obtained. And this method of impregnating the Buxton water with iron, muſt increaſe its tonic powers, and in many caſes improve its medicinal virtues. It is a common practice to join the uſe of a chalybeate ſpring, in the neighbourhood of St. Ann's well, with that of the Buxton water. But the ſuperiority of this artificial mineral water muſt be apparent, if we conſider its agreeable warmth, volatility, levity, and gratefulneſs to the palate.

Buxton bath is very frequently employed as a temperate cold bath. For as the heat of the water is ſixteen or eighteen degrees below that of the human body, a gentle ſhock is produced on the firſt immerſion, the heart and arteries are made to contract more powerfully, and the whole ſyſtem is braced and invigorated. But this ſalutary operation muſt be greatly diminiſhed, often indeed more than

than counterbalanced, by the relaxing vapours which copiously exhale from the bath, to which the patients are exposed during the time of dressing and undressing. A separate room is indeed provided for the ladies; but the gentlemen have no other accommodations than what the vault affords in which the bath is contained, and are therefore liable to all the inconveniences which arise from warmth and moisture.

June 12th, 1772. THE mercury in Farenheit's thermometer stood in the shade at 65; but in this vault quickly rose to 78 degrees.

EXPERIMENTS

ON

MATLOCK WATER.

EXPERIMENT I.

A Thermometer made by Dollond, and graduated according to Farenheit's ſcale, was expoſed for a ſufficient length of time to the ſtream of water as it guſhes out of the rock, and alſo immerſed in the baſon which receives it. The mercury roſe to 66 degrees.

EXPERIMENT II.

SIX drops of *ſp. ſal. ammon. vol.* were poured into a glaſs of the ſpring water, which

which contained about the ſixth of a pint; a very ſlight cloudineſs immediately enſued; but no precipitation was afterwards obſervable.

EXPERIMENT III.

Six drops of a ſolution of ſalt of tartar occaſioned a cloudineſs juſt perceptible, in the ſame quantity of water. No precipitation enſued.

EXPERIMENT IV.

Six drops of a ſolution of *ſaccharum ſaturni* immediately produced a milkineſs in the water, but no ſenſible precipitation.

EXPERIMENT V.

Six drops of a ſolution of ſilver in the nitrous acid inſtantly occaſioned a milkineſs in the water; and after ſtanding an hour, a grey powder was obſervable at the bottom of the glaſs.

EXPE-

EXPERIMENT VI.

TEN drops of the infuſion of galls neither produced any change of colour in the water at the time they were added, nor was the ſlighteſt purple hue perceptible two hours afterwards.

EXPERIMENT VII.

A PIECE of paper beſmeared with freſh ſyrup of violets was dipped into a glaſs full of water. No change of colour enſued.

EXPERIMENT VIII.

ANOTHER piece of paper, moiſtened in the ſame manner with the ſyrup, was placed over a glaſs of water, as ſoon as it was taken from the ſpring. The paper ſuffered no change of colour, although it remained an hour upon the glaſs.

EXPE-

EXPERIMENT IX.

My pulſe beat 84 ſtrokes in a minute at the time when I drank a half pint glaſs of the Matlock water. In twenty minutes my pulſe roſe to 88. In half an hour they ſunk to 82; and continued to vibrate the ſame number of times for an hour, which was as long as I thought it neceſſary to examine them.

EXPERIMENT X.

The mercury in Farenheit's thermometer, when immerſed in each of the baths ſtood at 68; in the river Derwent, which flows through the valley of Matlock, at 52. Theſe experiments were made on the 12th of June 1772, and the weather was warm.

EXPERIMENT XI.

A four once phial, after being accurately counterpoiſed in a very nice balance, was filled to the brim with diſtilled water, which weighed three ounces, four drachms, forty-five grains and a half. The ſame phial, exactly balanced as before, was then filled to the brim with Matlock water of the ſame temperature with the diſtilled water, which weighed three ounces, four drachms and forty-ſix grains.

Matlock water is grateful to the palate, and of an agreeable warmth, but exhibits no marks of any mineral ſpirit, either by its taſte, ſparkling appearance in the glaſs, or by the chemical teſt employed in experiment VIII. The ſecond and third experiments ſhew, that it is very ſlightly impregnated with *ſelenites*, or other earthy ſalts; and of this its comparative levity affords alſo a further proof. For it weighs twenty-ſix grains in a pint lighter than the Mancheſter pump water, *(a)* and only four grains heavier than diſtilled water.

(a) Vid. the Author's Treatiſe on the Pump Water of Mancheſter, Eſſays Medical and Experimental, p. 287, 2d. Edit.

water. The precipitation of a grey powder by the addition of a ſolution of ſilver in *aqua fortis* to the water, renders it probable that a ſmall portion of ſea ſalt is contained in it. For the powder is found to conſiſt of the particles of ſilver combined with the muriatic acid, which is ſeparated from the foſſil alkali by the ſuperior affinity the nitrous acid bears to it; and thus a double elective attraction takes place in this experiment.

THIS water has been ſaid to contain iron. But the aſſertion is at leaſt rendered doubtful by the ſixth experiment, which was made with the utmoſt accuracy; and I am inclined to think that it is entirely without foundation. The ſpring is juſtly celebrated for its efficacy in hæmoptoes; and hence it may have been too haſtily concluded that it poſſeſſes ſome ſlight degree of ſtypticity, by means of a chalybeate impregnation.

THE ninth experiment, which my ſhort

ſtay at Matlock would not allow me leiſure to repeat, affords a preſumption, that the water is not poſſeſſed of any ſtimulating powers. For the ſmall increaſe of quickneſs in my pulſe on drinking half a pint of it, may be aſcribed more to the qnantity received into the ſtomach, than to the heating quality of the water.

THE Briſtol and Matlock waters appear to reſemble each other both in their chemical and medicinal qualities. I have examined and compared them together by the teſts mentioned above; and ſo far as ſuch trials may be deemed concluſive, there ſeems to be no other than the following ſlight difference between them. The Briſtol water becomes a little more milky on the addition of a ſolution of fixed alkali, and of *ſaccharum ſaturni*, than that of Matlock. The former alſo weighs near a grain in a pint heavier than the latter. Is it not to be lamented therefore that ſo little attention is paid to Matlock, even by the Phyſicians who reſide in the neigh-

neighbourhood of it? In hectic cafes, hæmoptoes, the diabetes, and other diforders in which the circulation of the blood is rapid and irregular, I fhould apprehend that Matlock water, on fome accounts, claims the preference to that of Briftol. For as it is not fenfibly impregnated with any mineral fpirit, it fhould feem to be lefs difpofed to quicken the pulfe, and may therefore be drunk in larger quantities. But it muft be acknowledged that the climate of Briftol is fuperior to that of Matlock; a circumftance of the higheft importance to confumptive patients. Situated in a deep though delightful valley, and furrounded by very high mountains, the fun difappears at Matlock earlier in the evening, the fogs are longer in difperfing, and it may be prefumed that rain falls here more frequently and copioufly, than in other places. For at Chatfworth, which is encompaffed alfo with hills, and is about ten miles diftant, in 1764, 1765, 1767, and 1768, about thirty-three inches of rain at a medium fell each year.

THE following Table exhibits a comparative view of the different temperatures of Bath, Buxton, Briſtol, and Matlock waters, meaſured by Farenheit's thermometer.

*BATH.

King's Bath Pump	-	-	112°.
Hot Bath Pump	-	-	114½.
Croſs Bath Pump	-	-	110.

*BRISTOL.

Hot Well Pump	-	-	86.

BUXTON.

Bath	-	-	82.
St. Ann's Well	-	-	814.

MATLOCK.

Baths	-	-	68.
Spring	-	-	66.

* Vid. Mr. Canton's Experiments, Phil. Tranſ. vol. 57. page 203.

ON

ON THE
MEDICINAL USES
OF
FIXED AIR.

IN a courſe of experiments, which is yet too unfiniſhed to lay before the public, I have had frequent opportunities of obſerving that fixed air may, in no inconſiderable quantity, be breathed without danger or uneaſineſs. And it is a confirmation of this concluſion, that at Bath, where the waters copiouſly exhale this mineral ſpirit, (a) the bathers inſpire it

(a) See Dr. Falconer's very uſeful and ingenious Treatiſe on the Bath Waters, 2d. Edit. p. 313.

it with impunity. At Buxton alſo, where the bath is in a cloſe vault, the effects of ſuch *effluvia*, if noxious, muſt certainly be perceived.

Encouraged by theſe conſiderations, and ſtill more by the teſtimony of a very judicious Phyſician at Stafford in favour of this powerful antiſeptic remedy, I have adminiſtered fixed air in more than thirty caſes of the PHTHISIS PULMONALIS, by directing my patients to inſpire the ſteams of an efferveſcing mixture of chalk and vinegar, through the ſpout of a coffee-pot. The hectic fever has in ſeveral inſtances been conſiderably abated, and the matter expectorated has become leſs offenſive and better digeſted. I have not yet however been ſo fortunate in any one caſe, as to effect a cure; although the uſe of mephitic air has been accompanied with proper internal medicines. But Dr. Withering, the gentleman referred to above, informs me, that he has been more ſucceſsful. One phthiſical patient under his

his care, has by a ſimilar courſe entirely recovered; another was rendered much better; and a third, whoſe caſe was truly deplorable, ſeemed to be kept alive by it more than two months. It may be proper to obſerve, that fixed air can only be employed, with any proſpect of ſucceſs, in the latter ſtages of the *phthiſis pulmonalis,* when a purulent expectoration takes place. After the rupture and diſcharge of a VOMICA alſo, ſuch a remedy promiſes to be a powerful palliative. Antiſeptic fumigations and vapours have been long employed, and much extolled in caſes of this kind. I made the following experimont to determine whether their efficacy, in any degree, depends on the ſeparation of fixed air, from their ſubſtance.

ONE end of a bent tube was fixed in a phial full of lime water; the other end in a bottle of the tincture of myrrh. The junctures were carefully luted, and the phial containing the tincture of myrrh was

was placed in water, heated almoſt to the boiling point, by the lamp of a tea-kettle. A number of air bubbles were ſeparated, but probably not of the mephitic kind, for no precipitation enſued in the lime water. This experiment was repeated with the *tinct. tolutana, Ph. Ed.* and with *ſp. vinos. camph.* and the reſult was entirely the ſame. The medicinal action therefore of the vapours raiſed from ſuch tinctures, cannot be aſcribed to the extrication of fixed air; of which it is probable bodies are deprived by *chemical ſolution* as well as by *mixture.*

IF mephitic air be thus capable of correcting purulent matter in the lungs, we may reaſonably infer it will be equally uſeful when applied externally to foul ULCERS. And experience confirms the concluſion. Even the ſanies of a CANCER, when the carrot poultice failed, has been ſweetened by it, the pain mitigated, and a better digeſtion produced. The caſes I refer to are now in the Mancheſter Infirmary,

Infirmary, under the direction of my friend Mr. White, whofe fkill as a furgeon, and abilities as a writer are well known to the public.

Two months have elapfed fince thefe obfervations were written, (a) and the fame remedy, during that period, has been affiduoufly applied, but without any further fuccefs. The progrefs of the cancers feems to be checked by the fixed air; but it is to be feared, that a cure will not be effected. A palliative remedy, however, in a difeafe fo defperate and loathfome, may be confidered as a very valuable acquifition. Perhaps NITROUS AIR might be ftill more efficacious. This fpecies of factitious air is obtained from all the metals, except zinc, by means of the nitrous acid; and Dr. Prieftley informs me, that as a fweetener and antifeptic it far furpaffes fixed air. He put two mice into a quantity of it, one juft killed, the other offenfively putrid. After twenty-five days they were both perfectly fweet.

IN

(a) May, 1772.

In the ULCEROUS SORE THROAT much advantage has been experienced from the vapours of effervefcing mixtures, drawn into the *fauces*. (*a*) But this remedy fhould not fuperfede the ufe of other antifeptic applications. (*b*)

In MALIGNANT FEVERS, wines abounding with fixed air may be adminiftered, to check the feptic ferment, and fweeten the putrid *colluvies* in the *primæ viæ*. If the laxative quality of fuch liquors be thought an objection to the ufe of them, wines of a greater age may be given, impregnated with mephitic air, by a fimple but ingenious contrivance of my learned friend Dr. Prieftley, which will very foon be laid before the public. (*c*)

The

(*a*) Vid. Mr. White's ufeful Treatife on the Management of Pregnant and Lying-in Women, p. 279.

(*b*) See the Author's Obfervations on the efficacy of external applications in the Ulcerous Sore Throat, Effays Med. and Experimental, 2d. Edit. p. 377.

(*c*) DIRECTIONS for impregnating water with fixed air, in order to communicate to it the peculiar fpirit and virtues of Pyrmont water, and other mineral waters of a fimilar nature; by Jofeph Prieftley, L. L. D. F. R. S.

The patients common drink might alſo be medicated in the ſame way. A putrid *diarrhœa* frequently occurs in the latter ſtage of ſuch diſorders; and it is a moſt alarming and dangerous ſymptom. If the diſcharge be ſtopped by aſtringents a putrid *fomes* is retained in the body, which aggravates the delirium, and increaſes the fever. On the contrary, if it be ſuffered to take its courſe, the ſtrength of the patient muſt ſoon be exhauſted, and death unavoidably enſue. The injection of mephitic air into the inteſtines, under theſe circumſtances, bids fair to be highly ſerviceable. And a caſe of this deplorable kind has lately been communicated to me, in which the vapour of chalk and oil of vitriol, conveyed into the body, by the machine employed for tobacco clyſters, quickly reſtrained the *diarrhœa*, corrected the heat and fetor of the ſtools, and in two days removed every ſymptom of danger. A ſimilar inſtance of the ſalutary effects of mephitic air, thus adminiſtered, has occurred alſo in my my own practice; the hiſtory of which I ſhall probably lay before the public. May we not preſume that the ſame remedy would be equally uſeful in the DYSENTERY? The experiment is at leaſt worthy of trial.

THE uſe of wort, from its ſaccharine quality, and diſpoſition to ferment, has lately been propoſed as a remedy for the SEA SCURVY. Water, or other liquors already abounding with fixed air in a ſeparate ſtate, ſhould ſeem to be better adapted to this purpoſe, as they will more quickly correct the putrid diſpoſition of the fluids, and at the ſame time, by their gentle ſtimulus *(a)*, increaſe the powers of digeſtion, and give new ſtrength to the whole ſyſtem. Dr. Prieſtley, whoſe inventive genius ſuggeſted both the idea, and the means of executing it, has, under the ſanction of the College of Phyſicians, propoſed

(a) THE vegetables, which are moſt efficacious in the cure of the ſcurvy, poſſeſs ſome degree of a ſtimulating power.

propoſed the ſcheme to the Lords of the Admiralty, who have ordered trial to be made of it, on board ſome of his Majeſty's ſhips of war. Might it not, however, give additional efficacy to this remedy, if inſtead of ſimple water, the infuſion of malt were to be employed?

I AM perſuaded ſuch a medicinal drink might be preſcribed alſo with great advantage in ſcrophulous complaints, and other diſorders in which a general acrimony prevails, and the *craſis* of the blood is deſtroyed. Under ſuch circumſtances I have ſeen *vibices*, which ſpread over the body, diſappear in a few days, from the uſe of wort.

A GENTLEMAN, who is ſubject to a ſcorbutic eruption in his face, for which he has uſed a variety of remedies with no very beneficial effect, has lately applied the fumes of chalk and oil of vitriol to the parts affected. The operation occaſions great itching and prickling in the ſkin,

ſkin, and ſome degree of drowſineſs, but evidently abates the ſerous diſcharge, and diminiſhes the eruption. This patient has ſeveral ſymptoms which indicate a genuine ſcorbutic *diatheſis*; and it is probable that fixed air taken internally would be a uſeful medicine in his caſe.

THE ſaline draughts of Riverius are ſuppoſed to owe their antiemetic effects to the air, which is ſeparated from the ſalt of wormwood, during the act of effervescence. And the tonic powers of many mineral waters ſeem to depend on the ſame principle. But I ſhall exceed my deſign by enlarging further on this ſubject. What has been advanced, it is hoped, will ſuffice to excite the attention of Phyſicians to a remedy, which is capable of being applied to ſo many important medicinal purpoſes.

ON

On the antiseptic and sweetening powers, and on the varieties of FACTITIOUS AIR.

THOUGH the fact has lately been controverted by an ingenious writer, I am fully convinced with Dr. Macbride, from the evidence of repeated experiments, that fixed air has the property both of retarding and of correcting putrefaction. It may afford matter of amusement, to consider in what manner these effects are produced.

THAT fixed air may restrain, and even prevent putrefaction, without possessing any inherent antiseptic quality, is not difficult to conceive. For by surrounding the putrescent substance with that kind of air,

 which

which it yields by putrefaction, and which requires ſome vehicle to diſcharge or carry it off, the ſeparation of it is prevented, and the body thus retained in its original ſtate. This may be illuſtrated by a wet ſponge or cloth, which will never become dry in an atmoſphere ſaturated with moiſture. Or ſtill more appoſitely by putting a mixture of ſulphur and iron filings in a confined place, or in air in which candles have burned out. Under theſe circumſtances, no heat, effervefcence, or fume can be generated; whereas the ſame mixture in freſh air preſently grows hot, ſmokes copiouſly, and ſmells very offenſively. (a) The ſame obſervation will account for the curious fact mentioned by Dr. Alexander, that the *effluvia* of putrid ſubſtances retard putrefaction in the bodies expoſed to them. Perhaps, however, the generation of a volatile alkali may have ſome ſhare in producing this effect.

BUT

(a) See Doctor Prieſtley's moſt ingenious papers on factitious air, which will probably be publiſhed in the 62d. vol. of the Philoſophical Tranſactions.

But ſuppoſing the foregoing hypotheſis to be well founded, which I advance only as conjecture, how are we to explain the ſweetening powers of fixed air? An eminent philoſopher ſeems to hint that fixed air may act as a *menſtruum* for the putrid *effluvium*, and thus imbibe or diſcharge it from the ſeptic body. The ſame idea ſuggeſted itſelf to Mr. Henry, in conſequence of the following experiment, to which I was a witneſs. A piece of putrid fleſh was ſuſpended twelve hours, in a three pint bottle cloſely corked, and filled with fixed air, which had been ſeparated from chalk by the vitriolic acid. The beef was conſiderably ſweetened, but the air in the bottle was rendered intolerably offenſive. Now it affords a natural ſolution of this fact, if we admit that fixed air, by the laws of chemical affinity, abſtracts from the ſeptic body, and holds ſuſpended or diſſolved the putrid particles which it emits. And ſuch an affinity ſeems probable, from their ready combination, as well as from their diſpoſition to fly off together from putrefying ſubſtances. But how is the putrefactive proceſs checked, and the freſh generation of *effluvia* reſtrained under ſuch circumſtances? A piece of the ſame fleſh, which was employed in the foregoing experiment, was left all night in the external air, by the circulation of which the *effluvia* could not fail to be carried off as they were formed; yet the offenſive odour of the fleſh was not diminiſhed. Has not the reaſon of this difference, between the expoſure of a putrid ſubſtance to common air, and to mephitic air, been before aſſigned, when it was ſuggeſted that the latter may perhaps reſtrain the flight of that principle in bodies, the ſeparation of which conſtitutes an eſſential part of the proceſs of putrefaction? Animal fleſh will neither become putrid in *vacuo*, nor when cloſely confined from the acceſs of common air. In both caſes a vehicle is wanting for the eſcape of the mephitic air.

air. In like manner red hot wood ceases to burn, in inflammable air, because such air is already saturated with phlogiston.

I HAVE advanced the preceding conjectures, concerning the manner in which fixed air may retard and correct putrefaction, not as affording me full conviction, or to indulge a fanciful hypothesis, but to promote the further investigation of a subject so curious and interesting.

EXPERIMENT I.

IT is a fact lately ascertained by a very accurate Philosopher, that putrefaction generates air similar to that which animals have breathed. But this and the succeeding experiment shews that there is some little diversity in their properties and effects. Air was blown forcibly from the lungs, for a sufficient length of time, into a phial containing distilled water and iron filings. The water was then filtered, and a few drops of the infuſion of galls were added to it. A dark red colour, inclining to purple, was inſtantly produced.

*EXPERIMENT II.

Eight ounces of ox gall were poured into a bottle, which had a tube communicating with another phial, containing half an ounce of iron filings, and four ounces of diſtilled water. After ſtanding two days, part of the water was filtered, and ſuffered no change of colour from the addition of an aſtringent tincture. But the next day, when the fermentation in the gall was more evident, another filtered portion of the water ſtruck with the ſame tincture a deep roſy red. On the fifth and ſixth days, when the gall became intolerably putrid, though the vapour ſtill corroded the iron filings, it ſeemed to have loſt

* Communicated by Dr. Falconer of Bath.

loſt the power of diſſolving them. For the aſtringent tincture no longer produced any change of colour in the water, and the iron was evidently precipitated.

* EXPERIMENT III.

Solutions of iron in water, obtained by different kinds of fixed air, vary in the colours which they ſtrike with an infuſion of galls. When the vitriolic acid and foſſil alkali are employed, a black tinge is produced; when magneſia, or calcareous earths and the ſame acid are uſed, a purple hue is ſtruck; and when the air is ſupplied by fermentation, the artificial chalybeate is changed by galls into a roſy red.

EXPERIMENT IV.

Air diſcharged from chalk by the vitriolic acid readily and perfectly combines

* By the ſame.

with water; but when ſeparated by the nitrous acid, the union is more difficult to be effected, and much leſs complete. And the artificial mineral water, made by the latter, is more pungent and ſparkling than by the former acid.

EXPERIMENT V.

FACTITIOUS AIR, ſeparated from ſteel filings by the vitriolic acid, neither occaſioned any precipitation in lime water, nor rendered the cauſtic fixed alkali mild. Whereas the air ſet free from chalk and magneſia, by the ſame acid, inſtantly produced a milkineſs in lime water, and reſtored to the cauſtic alkali the power of efferveſcence.

EXPERIMENT VI.

A PIECE of putrid mutton, which had been employed as a ſtandard in ſome other experiments, was divided into two equal

equal parts: One of theſe was ſuſpended by a thread in a phial, containing an efferveſcing mixture of chalk and dilute ſpirit of vitriol; the other in a ſimilar phial, with a mixture of iron filings and the ſame acid. The mouths of the phials were ſlightly ſtopped with folded paper; and a briſk fermentation took place in each of them. After being expoſed ſixteen hours to the air detached from theſe ſubſtances, the bits of mutton were taken out, and examined. They were both conſiderably firmer in their texture; and the one which had been ſuſpended over the efferveſcing mixture of chalk and oil of vitriol was entirely ſweetened; but the putrid fetor of the other was not in the leaſt degree corrected.

EXPERIMENT VII.

A PIECE of putrid fleſh was ſuſpended about half an hour over a mixture of iron filings and nitrous acid, and was perfectly ly ſweetened. It had acquired a pungent and ſlightly acid ſmell, but remained firm and free from fetor when this odour was waſhed off. The water, in which the fleſh was waſhed, did not efferveſce with *lixivium tartari*; nor did the vapour ariſing from the ſpirit of nitre and iron filings produce any change of colour in a paper covered with ſyrup of violets; preſumptive proofs that the ſweetneſs of the fleſh was not reſtored by any acid fumes.

THE fixed air of metals ſeems, by ſome of theſe experiments, to be of a kind different from that which is contained in alkalis and calcareous earths. And conſequently the action of theſe ſubſtances as *fluxes*, cannot be explained on the principle of their reſtoring the air which had been loſt by calcination. Indeed there are other proofs that the reſuſcitation of calces does not depend on this cauſe. I have been aſſured by an able Chemiſt that he has repeatedly reſtored *minium* to

its

its metalline ſtate, by the cauſtic alkali, aſſiſted by a proper degree of heat; and that ſeveral of the metals may be revived by the force of fire alone. It is true that a mild calcareous earth employed as a flux, is always rendered cauſtic by the operation. But this may be owing to the action of the fire, and not to the loſs of its air by elective attraction. Perhaps the operation of alkalis and calcareous earths as fluxes may depend on their abſorbing the matter which ſeems to be added to metallic ſubſtances by the proceſs of calcination, and which furniſhes ſuch an amazing increaſe of weight *(a)*? Inflammable bodies may produce the ſame effect, by volatilizing and carrying it off.

(a) ANTIMONY, when calcined, gains one eleventh part of its original weight; zinc one tenth; tin one ſixth; and lead, when converted into minium, one fourth.

* ON THE NOXIOUS VAPOURS OF CHARCOAL.

—— *Sævamque exhala opacat mephitim.*
Virgil. Æneid. lib. 7. 34.

THE accurate and ingenious Doctor Hales, has proved by a great variety of experiments, that air enters in a very considerable proportion into the composition of all bodies. That air thus combined, is in a fixed state, and contributes to form the union and firm connection of the constituent parts of bodies; and

* Communicated by Dr. Dobson of Liverpool.

and that on their destruction or decomposition, this fixed air is again restored to its state of elasticity.

Fixed air, whether procured by fire, fermentation, or chemical resolution, has been supposed to be a body *sui generis*; and to possess properties, by which it is always distinctly characterised. It is more comformable however to the simplicity which is constantly observed in the operations of nature, to conclude, that as it is common atmospheric air which enters into the composition of bodies, it is likewise the same air which is again detached, on their decomposition or destruction; that its varieties depend on adventitious matter; and that it has different degrees of mixture and composition, according as it is obtained from different substances, or by a different process.

That by degrees however, it is decompounded; returns to its original simplicity;

plicity; is reſtored to the common magazine from which it was taken; and that the atmoſphere is thus conſtantly gaining by one proceſs, what it loſes by another.

Factitious or fixed air is the general term, by which this ſubject is diſtinguiſhed; and when it produces any noxious effects, either in conſequence of the proceſs by which it is procured, or the manner in which it is applied, it may then be properly called mephitic air.

Much has been done by ſome very ingenious modern writers, to illuſtrate this ſubject; and much ſtill remains to be done, to compleat the chemical and medical hiſtory of fixed air. The preſent commentary, chiefly reſpects the factitious air of charcoal; or the mephitic vapours which ariſe from this ſubſtance, in the ſtate of ignition. And the following hiſtory points out both the noxious qualities of theſe vapours, and their mode of action on the animal œconomy.

October

October 5th, 1769. A ſervant to a gentleman's family in Liverpool, ſhut himſelf up in a ſmall room to clean plate. In this room there was a chafing-diſh of burning charcoal, and the door and window were cloſed. He ſoon felt himſelf *very ill*, as he expreſſed it; was chilly, ſickiſh, and had ſhooting pains in the head. He continued to be affected in this manner for upwards of an hour and a half, during which time he had been twice called out, but returned again to the ſame ſituation in a few minutes. The chills, ſickneſs, and pain in the head became more ſevere, and were increaſed by fits; he retched, but could not vomit. Theſe were the only ſenſations he could recollect; and on my aſking him, whether he did not feel an oppreſſion at his breaſt, or a ſenſe of ſuffocation, he anſwered in the negative.

He remembered that he heard the clock ſtrike eleven, which was an hour and

and a half from his firſt going into the room; and ſtill finding himſelf very ill, but having no ſuſpicion of the cauſe, he leaned forwards, reſted his head upon his hands, and from that time had no further knowledge of what paſſed.

About half an hour after this, ſome of the family going near the door, were alarmed by his groans. The door was forced open, and he was found extended on the ground; his eyes fixed and ſtaring; his hands clenched; his arms, legs, and whole body rigid; and his countenance, which was naturally pale, had now a death-like appearance.

He was immediately carried into the open air; but it was with difficulty that his limbs were ſo bent that he could be ſeated in a chair. He continued to groan, and on the application of hartſhorn drops to his noſe, exerted a kind of motion, as if offended. Cold water thrown upon his face,

face, had a more powerful effect to rouse him. After ten minutes, he came to himself; and in about twenty minutes, he was able to walk.

At this time I first saw him; he complained of pain in his head, coldness and sickness; was hot to the touch; his pulse, small and frequent, 120 in a minute. While I was examining him, I observed his voice faultered; his eyes became fixed; he staggered forwards, and would have fallen, had he not been supported. He was placed in a chair, and remained in a state of insensibility near a minute; there was no rigidity, the colour of the countenance did not change, but the pulse was extremely small, frequent, and irregular. On coming to himself, he complained much of pain in his head, was sick, retched, trembled, and was cold and hot by fits; a considerable degree of fever remained for two days, and then gradually left him.

We have here a fair opportunity of obſerving the effects of theſe noxious vapours. The patient was near two hours ſtruggling with the poiſon; and the whole progreſs of the ſymptoms clearly points out, an immediate affection of the brain and nervous ſyſtem, not of the lungs.

It is the common apprehenſion, that thoſe who are killed by the effluvia of burning charcoal, are *ſuffocated*; and this apprehenſion is ſupported by the authorities of ſome very diſtinguiſhed practical writers.

Morgagni, in his excellent work *de Sedibus et Cauſis Morborum*, aſſerts, that thoſe who die from the *ſteams of charcoal*, the ſteams of the fermenting grape, in the Grotto di Cani, and in the cavern of Pyrmont, are *ſuffocated*. *(a)*

Hoffman, in his Diſſertation *de fumo carbonum*

(a) Epiſt. 19. §. 40.

carbonum noxio, ſays, that theſe vapours being received into the breaſt, diſtend the lungs, prevent the admiſſion of air, and thus *ſuffocate.* (*b*) The mode of operation is expreſſed in very ſtrong terms. *Eadem enim horum operandi ratio eſt, ac ſi aſperam arteriam filo conſtringas; nam utroque horum aeris ſufficiens introitus impeditur.* (*c*)

Doctor Hales concludes, that the ſteams of the Grotto di Cani, and ſeveral other noxious vapours, deſtroy the elaſticity of the air, occaſion the veſicles of the lungs to collapſe, and thus *ſuffocate,* and cauſe ſudden death. (*d*)

Such are the reſpectable authorities which give weight to the common opinion, that thoſe who are killed by theſe noxious effluvia, are ſuffocated. The following experiments, hiſtories, and ob-

 ſervations,

(*b*) Hoffman, tom. 4. p. 697. 22. (*c*) Ib.

(*d*) Hale's Statics. p. 260, 261.

ſervations tend, however, to eſtabliſh a different doctrine.

We learn from the experiments of the celebrated Greenwood, that the air of a well, in which the men who went down periſhed, and in which a lighted torch was inſtantly extinguiſhed, did not differ from common air, either in gravity, humidity, or elaſticity. *(e)*

The ſame is found to be true of the Grotto di Cani. In this, the height of the mercury in the barometer was not altered by the deadly vapours. *(f)* And we have the ſame proof of the ſtate of the air in the cavern of Pyrmont. *(g)* It appears likewiſe from the experiments of the learned Leonardo Capuano, that thoſe animals which do *not breath*, are deſtroyed in the Grotto di Cani, though ſlowly and with more difficulty.*

Doctor

(e) Saggio delle Tranſar. tom. 5. p. 2.

(f) Mead. de Venenis, tent. 6.

(g) Commerc. litter. A. 1737. Heb. 8.

* Delle Moſette, Lez. 1.

DOCTOR HALES indeed proves, that the fumes of burning ſulphur, and the exhalations from the lungs of animals, bring into a fixed ſtate part of the air through which they are diſperſed, and conſequently diminiſh its elaſticity. That this circumſtance however is not the cauſe of death, is hence evident; in high winds and ſtorms, and on aſcending very high mountains, a greater diminution of elaſticity takes place, without ſuch fatal effects. †

ALL theſe noxious vapours, whether ariſing from burning charcoal, the fermenting grape, the Grotti di Cani, or the cavern of Pyrmont, operate nearly in the ſame manner. When accumulated and confined, their effects are often inſtantaneous; they immediately deſtroy the action of the brain and nerves, and in a moment arreſt the vital motions. When

† Veratti Com. Acad. Bonon. tom. ii. Pt. II. p. 271. 276, And Element. Phyſiolog. Haller. vol. 3. p. 208.

more diffuſed, their effects are ſlower, but ſtill evidently mark out a direct affection of the nervous ſyſtem.

THOSE who are expoſed to the vapours of the fermenting grape, are as inſtantly deſtroyed, as they would be by the ſtrongeſt electrical ſhock. A ſtate of inſenſibility is the immediate effect upon thoſe animals which are thruſt into the Grotti di Cani, or the cavern of Pyrmont; the animal is deprived of motion, lies as if dead, and if not quickly returned into the freſh air, is irrecoverable. And if we attend to the hiſtories of thoſe who have ſuffered from the vapours of burning charcoal, we ſhall in like manner find, that the brain and moving powers, are the parts primarily affected.

A COOK who had been accuſtomed to make uſe of lighted charcoal more than his buſineſs required, and to ſtand with his head over theſe fires, complained

for

for a year of very acute pain in the head; and after this, was ſeized with a paralytic affection of the lower limbs, and a ſlow fever. *(h)*

A PERSON was left reading in bed with a pan of charcoal in a corner of the room. On being viſited early the next morning, he was found with his eyes ſhut, his book open and laid on one ſide, his candle extinguiſhed, and to appearance like one in a deep ſleep. Stimulants and cupping glaſſes gave no relief; but he was ſoon recovered by the free acceſs of freſh air. *(i)*

FOUR priſoners, in order to make their eſcape, attempted to deſtroy the iron work of their windows, by the means of burning charcoal. As ſoon as they commenced their operations, the fumes of the charcoal being confined by the cloſeneſs of the priſon, one of them was ſtruck dead;

H 4 another

(h) Morgagni. Epiſt. 64. §. 15. *(i)* Cheſneau, 696.

another was found pale, ſpeechleſs, and without motion; afterwards he ſpoke incoherently, was ſeized with a fever and died. The other two were with great difficulty recovered. (k)

Two boys went to warm themſelves in a ſtove heated with charcoal. In the morning they were found deſtitute of ſenſe and motion, with countenances as compoſed as in a placid ſleep. There were ſome remains of pulſe, but they died in a ſhort time. (l)

A FISHERMAN depoſited a large quantity of charcoal in a deep cellar. Some time afterwards, his ſon, a healthy ſtrong man, went down into the cellar with a pan of burning charcoal and a light in his hand. He had ſcarcely deſcended to the bottom, when his candle went out. He returned, lighted his candle, and again deſcended. Soon

(k) Donatus Epiſt. 694. (l) Ib. 695.

Soon after he called aloud for aſſiſtance. His mother, brother, and a ſervant haſted to give him relief, but none of them returned. Two others of the village ſhared the ſame fate. It was then determined to throw large quantities of water into the cellar; and after two or three days, they had acceſs to the dead bodies.*

Cælius Aurelianus ſays, that thoſe who are injured by the fumes of charcoal, become cataleptic. *(m)* And Hoffman himſelf, in another part of his works, enumerates a train of ſymptoms which in no reſpect correſpond with his idea of ſuffocation. Thoſe who ſuffer from the fumes of burning charcoal, ſays he, have ſevere pains in the head, great debility, faintneſs, ſtupor and lethargy. *(n)*

It appears from the above hiſtories and obſervations, that theſe vapours exert their

* Hiſtoire de l' Academié de ſcience, Ann. 1710.

(m) De morbis acutis, lib. ii. c. x.

(n) Tom. 1. p. 229. § 5.

their noxious effects on the brain and nerves. Sometimes they occasion sudden death; at other times, the various symptoms of a debilitated nervous system, according as the poison is more or less concentrated. The olfactory nerves are first and principally affected, and the brain and nervous system by sympathy or consent of parts. It is well known, that there is a strong and ready consent between the olfactory nerves and many other parts of the nervous system. The effluvia of flowers and perfumes, in delicate or irritable habits, produce a train of symptoms, which though transient, are analogous to those which are produced by the vapours of charcoal; viz. vertigo, sickness, faintness, and sometimes a total insensibility. The female malefactor, whom Doctor Mead inoculated by putting into the nostrils dossils of cotton impregnated with variolous matter, was immediately on the introduction, afflicted with a most excruciating head ach, and had a constant fever till after the eruption.

THE

The vapours of burning charcoal, and other poiſonous effluvia, frequently produce their prejudicial and even fatal effects, without being either offenſive to the ſmell, or oppreſſive to the lungs. It is a matter of importance therefore, that the common opinion ſhould be more agreeable to truth; for where ſuffocation is ſuppoſed to be the effect, there will be little apprehenſion of danger, ſo long as the breaſt keeps free from pain or oppreſſion.

It may be well to remember, that the poiſon itſelf is diſtinct from that groſs matter which is offenſive to the ſmell; and that this is frequently in its moſt active ſtate, when undiſtinguiſhed by the ſenſe. Were the following cautions generally attended to, they might in ſome inſtances be the happy means of preſerving life. Never to be confined with burning charcoal in a ſmall room, or where there is not a free draught of air by by a chimney or ſome other way. Never to venture into any place in which air has been long pent up, or which from other circumſtances ought to be ſuſpected; unleſs ſuch ſuſpected place be either previouſly well ventilated, or put to the teſt of the lighted candle. For it is a ſingular and well known fact, that the life of flame, is in ſome circumſtances ſooner affected and more expeditiouſly extinguiſhed by noxious vapours, than animal life. A proof of which I remember to have received from a very intelligent Clergyman, who was preſent at a muſical entertainment in the theatre at Oxford. The theatre was crouded; and during the entertainment, the candles were obſerved to burn dim, and ſome of them went out. The audience complained only of faintneſs and languor; but had the animal effluvia been ſtill further accumulated or longer confined, they would have been extinguiſhed as well as the candles.

The most obvious, effectual, and expeditious means of relief to those who have unhappily suffered from this cause, are such as will dislodge and wash away the poison, restore the energy of the brain and nerves, and renew the vital motions. Let the patient therefore be immediately carried into the open air, and let the air be fanned backwards and forwards to assist its action; let cold water be thrown on the face, and let the face, mouth and nostrils be repeatedly washed; and as soon as practicable get the patient to drink some cold water. But if the case is too far gone to be thus relieved, let a healthy person breathe into the mouth of the patient; and gently force air into the mouth, throat and nostrils. Frictions, cupping, bleeding, and blisters are likewise indicated. And if after the instant danger is removed, a fever be excited, the method of cure must be adapted to the nature and prevailing symptoms of the fever.

ON THE

ATRABILIS.

THE ancients, as appears from Galen, ſuppoſed the *atrabilis* to be derived either from the dregs of the blood, or from yellow bile torrefied and highly concocted. A celebrated modern anatomiſt is of opinion that it is blood, which having lodged ſome time in the inteſtinal canal, has acquired a blackneſs and putridity. But is it not more probable that in general it is no other than gall, become acrid by ſtagnation in the *veſica fellea*, and rendered viſcid by the abſorption of its fluid parts? When diſcharged into the *duodenum* in this ſtate, it occaſions univerſal diſturb-

diſturbance and diſorder, till evacuated either by vomiting or purging. I have lately had under my care a young gentleman, labouring under a *maraſmus*, produced by exceſſive intemperance. During the courſe of his diſorder, which at laſt proved fatal, he ſeveral times voided both by ſtool and vomiting, a conſiderable quantity of black, tenacious, and moſt offenſive bile. The ſymptoms preceding the diſcharge, and which ceaſed ſoon afterwards, were a quick pulſe, head ach, delirium, hiccup, intenſe thirſt, inward heat, and an uncommon fœtor in his breath. A lady aged thirty, unhappily addicted to habits which have a peculiarly pernicious effect upon the liver, after a conſtipation of the belly during ſix days, was ſeized with a violent and inceſſant vomiting of black and viſcid bile. The *infuſum ſenæ limoniatum*, warmed with the tincture of Columbo ſoon checked her reachings, and operating by ſtool prevented the return of her vomiting. The matter

ter diſcharged in both theſe caſes bore not the leaſt reſemblance to grumous blood. I have ſeveral times obſerved the febrile ſymptoms in children, which are aſcribed to dentition, relieved by theſe pitchy ſtools. And I recollect three caſes of the *acute aſthma*, as Dr. Millar terms it, the paroxyſms of which ſeemed to be critically terminated by a ſimilar evacuation. Whether in theſe inſtances the black bile was the cauſe or the effect of the diſeaſe, cannot with certainty be determined; but the former appears to be the more probable opinion.

ON THE SEPTIC QUALITY OF SEA SALT, &c. &c.

SIR JOHN PRINGLE obſerves that one drachm of ſea ſalt preſerves two drachms of freſh beef, in two ounces of water, above thirty hours uncorrupted, in a heat equal to that of the human body, that is twenty hours longer than water alone; but that half a drachm of ſalt does not preſerve it above two hours longer than pure water; that twenty-five grains have little or no antiſeptic virtue; and that ten

 grains

grains both heighten and haſten the corruption of the fleſh. *(a)* The reſult of this experiment is ſo curious and unexpected, that I wiſhed to aſcertain the cauſe of it.

EXPERIMENT I.

May 15th, 1772. EQUAL parts, viz. two drachms of the lean of mutton, chopped very ſmall, were ſeparately put into five wide mouthed phials, and to each were added two ounces of pump water. Ten grains of ſea ſalt were diſſolved in the firſt; the ſame quantity of brown bay ſalt in the ſecond; of *ſal cathartícus amarus* in the third; and of true glauber's ſalt in the fourth. The fifth contained only fleſh and water, and was intended for a ſtandard. The bottles were ſlightly corked, and after a gentle agitation placed in a window, expoſed to the weſtern ſun. The mercury in Farenheit's thermometer then ſtood in the ſhade at 65 degrees.

IN

(a) Pringle's Diſeaſes of the Army, Appendix, p. 38.

In twenty-nine hours the mixture which contained the *ſal catharticus amarus* had acquired ſomewhat of a putrid taint.

In forty hours the ſtandard was ſlightly offenſive. The mixture with ſea ſalt was putrid, and that with the cathartic ſalt was yet more putrid.

In fifty hours the ſtandard and the two mixtures above-mentioned were equally putrid. The two others were ſweet.

In ſixty-two hours the ſtandard was become much more offenſively putrid than the two mixtures with ſea ſalt, and cathartic ſalt, in which the putrefactive proceſs appeared not to have advanced any further. The fleſh with the brown bay ſalt was now ſlightly tainted; but that with the true glauber's ſalt was ſtill ſweet.

In ſeventy-five hours the mixture with brown bay ſalt was become putrid, and that with the true glauber's ſalt a little offenſive. And in twelve hours longer the latter mixture was alſo putrid.

FROM this experiment it appears that common ſalt, in the quantity of ten grains promotes putrefaction, and that the *ſal catharticus amarus* in the ſame proportion is yet more ſeptic; but that bay ſalt in this quantity reſiſts putrefaction, and that true glauber's ſalt exceeds in this reſpect even bay ſalt. The ſeptic and antiſeptic qualities of theſe ſalts, when uſed in ſo minute a quantity, are therefore evidently dependent on, and proportioned to their degrees of purity. Alimentary ſalt, it is well known, contains in its cryſtals an earthy ſalt, ſimilar to that of Epſom; which is a powerful ferment, almoſt equally capable in a ſmall as in a large quantity, of exciting the putrefactive proceſs in ſubſtances diſpoſed to it. Whereas the pure neutral itſelf, which conſiſts of the muriatic acid and the foſſil alkali, can only exert its antiſeptic powers when uſed in a proportion adequate

adequate to the action of the bitter salt with which it is combined, and superiour to the putrid tendency of the animal flesh, which it is employed to preserve. (b)

EXPERIMENT II.

May 21. Six days from the commencement of the experiment, the pieces of flesh in the solutions of common salt, and of *sal catharticus amarus*, were not more offensive than on the third day; and the mixtures emitted no air bubbles. But the standard at this time was intolerably putrid, very frothy, and the bits of mutton had risen to the surface of the water.

This experiment shews that both sea salt and the bitter purging salt, though they quicken putrefaction, prevent the progress of it beyond a certain degree. A quality which

(b) Sir John Pringle informs me, he has long suspected, but never ascertained the fact by experiment, that the septic quality of sea salt is owing to some heterogeneous substance joined to it.

which muſt increaſe the uſefulneſs of the former, as a ſeaſoning to our food.

A LATE eminent and learned writer has related the hiſtory of a violent ſcurvy, produced by drinking ſea water. A young lady, aged 16, tall, thin, and of a delicate conſtitution, though in tolerable good health, was adviſed to uſe ſea water on account of a ſtrumous ſwelling and inflammation of her upper lip. She drank a pint of it every morning for ten days ſucceſſively; which did not paſs off freely by the uſual evacuations. At the end of this period ſhe was ſuddenly ſeized with a profuſe diſcharge of the *catamenia*, was perpetually ſpitting blood from the gums, and had innumerable petechial ſpots on different parts of her body. Her pulſe was quick, though full; her face pale and ſomewhat bloated; and her fleſh ſoft and tender. She was often faint, but ſoon recovered her ſpirits. The flux from the *uterus* at length abated; but that from the gums increaſed to ſuch a degree, that

her

her Apothecary took a little blood from her arm. From the orifice blood continually ouzed for ſeveral days. At laſt an hœmorrhage from the noſe came on, attended with frequent faintings, in which ſhe at length expired, choaked as it were with her own blood. Before ſhe died, her right arm was mortified from the elbow to the wriſt. And it is further to be remarked, that though blood let from her ſome weeks before ſhe began the uſe of ſea water, was ſufficiently denſe; yet that drawn in her laſt ſickneſs was mere putrid, and diſſolved gore. (a)

DOCTOR HUXHAM explains the diſſolvent action of ſea water in this inſtance, by ſuppoſing an accumulation of the marine ſalt in the maſs of blood, which running into *moleculæ*, too large to paſs the minuteſt veſſels, occaſioned ſtagnations; and by irritating the capillaries, produced ruptures of them, extravaſations, blotches, and livid ſpots. But do not the preceding ex-

 periments

(a) Vid. Philoſ. Tranſact. Vol. 53, p. 6.

periments ſuggeſt a better ſolution of the fact? Sea water abounds with the cathartic ſalt, which conſtitutes the bittern of it; and this has been proved to be a powerful ſeptic.

A PHYSICIAN who often takes magneſia, to correct an acidity in his ſtomach, ariſing from indigeſtion, invariably obſerves that the diſcharges which it produces are peculiarly putrid and offenſive. Hence it is probable that this earth combined with an acid of the vegetable as well as of the mineral claſs, promotes putrefaction. Should we not therefore employ the *ſal catharticus amarus* and *magneſia alba* with caution, in diſeaſes of a putrid tendency?

I CANNOT omit this opportunity of recommending the calcination of magneſia, as a great improvement of that medicine. The loſs of its fixed air, which by this proceſs appears to conſtitute ſeven twelfths of of its weight, obviates the flatulence which it produces in the *primæ viæ*, without diminiſhing its purgative or abſorbent qualities. Care however ſhould be taken that the magneſia be free from any calcareous earth, otherwiſe the action of the fire will render this mild powder offenſively cauſtic to the ſtomach, as I have more than once experienced. Magneſia may be calcined with very little trouble, in a common crucible placed in a glowing fire, and kept red hot during the ſpace of two hours. This improvement was ſuggeſted to me by a Phyſician in London, diſtinguiſhed for his knowledge of chemiſtry.

ON

ON

COFFEE.

THOUGH coffee has been in general uſe for more than a century paſt, has been analyſed by fire, and variouſly inveſtigated by writers of learning and reputation; yet neither chemiſtry nor experience have hitherto aſcertained its true nature, or medicinal qualities. Of this the contradictory teſtimonies which have been delivered concerning it, afford a painful evidence. For it is ſurely to be lamented that an article of diet, active in its powers, and univerſally employed, ſhould

ſhould be ſo little underſtood. The following experiments may perhaps lead to farther enquiries on this uſeful ſubject.

EXPERIMENT I.

THIRTY berries of roaſted, and the ſame number of unroaſted coffee were each digeſted, forty-eight hours, in two ounces of rectified ſpirit of wine. The former tincture was ſtrongly impregnated with the peculiar taſte and odour of the coffee; the latter had acquired little or no ſenſible flavour.

EXPERIMENT II.

TEN drops of a ſolution of green vitriol, were added to a tea ſpoonful of each of the above-mentioned tinctures, diluted with an ounce of water. Both aſſumed a purple colour; but the change was greateſt in the tincture prepared with unroaſted coffee.

A ſi-

A ſimilar difference was obſervable in the infuſions of roaſted and unroaſted coffee prepared with water, allowance being made for the dark hue communicated to the *menſtruum* by the roaſted coffee.

These facts evince the action of fire in diminiſhing aſtringency; and furniſh an additional proof of the impropriety of employing heat in preparations of the bark, and other vegetables of a like quality. (a)

EXPERIMENT III.

Two drachms of roaſted mutton chopped very ſmall, were digeſted in an ounce of pump water, and in the ſame quantity of a ſtrong infuſion of roaſted coffee. The phials which contained the mixtures, were placed at a moderate diſtance

(a) Vid. the Author's Eſſays Medical and Experimental, 2d. edit.

tance from the fire, ſo as to be kept nearly blood warm. In thirty hours the mutton and water became putrid; but the infuſion of coffee continued ſweet twelve hours longer.

EXPERIMENT IV.

To aſcertain the action of coffee on the digeſtion of food in the ſtomach, I prepared three alimentary mixtures, conſiſting of equal parts, viz. two drachms of roaſted mutton, of the crumb of bread, and of ſaliva, beat into a pulp, and ſeverally combined with an ounce of the infuſions of coffee, of green tea, and the ſame quantity of pump water. The bottles were placed (as in the former experiment) at a proper diſtance from the fire, and every now and then carefully examined. A fermentation was firſt perceived in the ſtandard, i. e. the mixture with pump water, which became ſour in about forty-eight

eight hours. The infuſion of coffee emitted few air bubbles, and continued near four days without ſhewing any ſigns of acidity. By an accident, the phial which contained the tea was broken at the beginning of the experiment.

EXPERIMENT V.

March 29th, 1772. I awoke at five o'clock in the morning with the head-ach. My pulſe was hard and full, and beat 92 ſtrokes in a minute. I drank four diſhes of ſtrong coffee. In half an hour the pain in my head was relieved; yet my pulſe ſtill continued to vibrate the ſame number of times, but was ſofter and leſs full. In an hour it ſunk to 70. In an hour and a half it roſe again to 76; and in two hours to 80, which is the ſtandard of its frequency in health. I was in a recumbent poſture during the whole time of this experiment, which I have

have ſince repeated ſeveral times, under different circumſtances, with no material variation in the reſult.

FROM theſe obſervations we may infer that coffee is ſlightly aſtringent, and antiſeptic; that it moderates alimentary fermentation, and is powerfully ſedative. Its action on the nervous ſyſtem probably depends on the oil it contains; which receives its flavour, and is rendered mildly empyreumatic by the proceſs of roaſting: Neumann obtained by diſtillation from one pound of coffee, five ounces, five drachms and a half of water; ſix ounces and half a drachm of thick fœtid oil, and four ounces and two drachms of a *caput mortuum*. And it is well known that rye, torrefied with a few almonds, which furniſh the neceſſary proportion of oil, is now frequently employed as a ſubſtitute for theſe berries.

The MEDICINAL QUALITIES of coffee ſeem to be derived from the grateful ſenſation

ſation which it produces in the ſtomach; and from the ſedative powers it exerts on the *vis vitæ*. Hence it aſſiſts digeſtion, and relieves the head-ach; and is taken in large quantities, with peculiar propriety, by the Turks and Arabians, becauſe it counteracts the narcotic effects of opium, to the uſe of which thoſe nations are much addicted.

In delicate habits it often occaſions watchfulneſs, tremors, and many of thoſe complaints which are denominated nervous. It has even been ſuſpected of producing palſies, and from my own obſervation I ſhould apprehend, not entirely without foundation. Slare affirms that he became paralytic by the too liberal uſe of coffee; and that his diſorder was removed by abſtinence from that liquor.

Coffee berries are ſaid to be remarkably diſpoſed to imbibe exhalations from other bodies, and thereby to acquire an adven-

adventitious and disagreeable flavour. A bottle of rum placed at some distance from a canister of coffee, so impregnated the berries in a short time as to injure their flavour. Some years since a few bags of pepper were conveyed in a coffee-ship from India, the effluvia of which being absorbed by the coffee, the whole cargo was spoiled. (a)

(a) Miller's Gardener's Dictionary, 8th. Edition, Article, COFFEE.

A REVIEW OF THE MOST IMPORTANT CONCLUSIONS DEDUCED FROM THE PRECEDING EXPERIMENTS.

1. COLUMBO ROOT yields its virtues moſt perfectly to rectified ſpirit of wine; and to other *menſtrua* in the following order. 1. To French brandy. 2. to Madeira wine. 3. to white wine. 4. to diſtilled water. 5. to white wine vinegar. 6. to hard pump water.

2. THE watery infuſion of Columbo root is more periſhable than that of other bitters. In twenty-four hours a copious precipitation takes place in it; and in two days it becomes ropy, and even muſty.

3. THE

3. The addition of orange peel renders the infuſion of Columbo root leſs ungrateful to the palate.

4. Twelve ounces of Columbo root yield eight ounces and two drachms of extract, which retains the entire flavour of the root, and is equal, if not ſuperiour in efficacy to the powder.

5. Peruvian bark reſiſts the putrefaction of animal fleſh more powerfully than the Columbo root; but as a preſervative of the bile from putridity, this root exceeds the cortex.

6. Peruvian bark mixed with putrid gall, inſtantly produces a coagulation, and conſiderably increaſes the fœtor of it. Whereas the infuſion of Columbo root unites perfectly with it, and very powerfully corrects its offenſive ſmell. This ſerves in ſome meaſure to explain the ac-

 tion

tion of this remedy in the *cholera morbus*, and other diſeaſes attended with a redundance and depravation of the bile.

7. COLUMBO ROOT moderates, without ſuſpending the fermentation of alimentary mixtures; prevents them from growing ſour; and neutraliſes acidities when formed, much more completely than Peruvian bark, or chamomile flowers.

8. COLUMBO ROOT does not increaſe the quickneſs of the pulſe; and may therefore be uſed with propriety in the *pthiſis pulmonalis*, and in hectical caſes, to correct acrimony, and to ſtrengthen the organs of digeſtion.

9. THE Columbo root is a uſeful remedy in the *cholera morbus*; in diarrhœas; in the dyſentery; in bilious fevers; in a languid ſtate of the ſtomach, attended with want of appetite, nauſea, and indigeſtion; and in habitual vomitings, when they

they proceed from a weakneſs or irritability of the ſtomach, from an irregular gout, from acidities, or from acrimonious bile.

10. The ORCHIS ROOT might be cultivated to great advantage in England, and SALEP which is a preparation of it, might be afforded at eight-pence or ten-pence per pound. Whereas foreign ſalep is now ſold at five or ſix ſhillings per pound.

11. RICE, as an aliment, is inferior to ſalep; being ſlow of fermentation, and a very weak corrector of putrefaction. It is therefore an improper diet for hoſpital patients; and more particularly for ſailors, in long voyages; becauſe it ſeems incapable of preventing, and will not contribute much to check the progreſs of that fatal diſeaſe the ſea ſcurvy.

12. CHEESE, when mellowed by age, ferments readily with fleſh and water;

 but

but ſeparates a rancid oil, which appears to be incapable of any further change, and muſt, as a ſeptic, be pernicious in the ſcurvy. The ſame objection may be urged, with ſtill greater propriety, againſt the uſe of cheeſe in hoſpitals; becauſe convaleſcents are ſo liable to relapſes, that the ſlighteſt error of diet may occaſion them.

13. Salep has the ſingular property of concealing the taſte of ſalt water; a circumſtance of the higheſt importance at ſea, when there is a ſcarcity of freſh water.

14. Salep retards the acetous fermentation of milk; and conſequently would be a good lithing for milk pottage, eſpecially in large towns, where the cattle being fed upon ſour draft, muſt yield aceſcent milk.

15. Salep, in a certain proportion, would be a uſeful and profitable addition to

to bread. For by abſorbing and retaining more water than flour alone is capable of, it occaſions a conſiderable increaſe of weight.

16. BUXTON WATER is found, by analyſis, to contain calcareous earth, foſſil alkali, and ſea ſalt; but in very ſmall proportions. For a gallon of the water, when evaporated, yields only twenty-four grains of ſediment.

17. THE temperature of Buxton bath is 82 degrees of Farenheit's thermometer; that of St. Ann's well ſomewhat leſs.

18. BUXTON water, when drunk, quickens the pulſe very conſiderably, and ſometimes occaſions the head-ach. By the ſixed air which it contains, it readily diſſolves iron; and ſuch an impregnation muſt, in many caſes, improve its medicinal virtues.

19. MATLOCK WATER is grateful to the palate, and of an agreeable warmth, but exhibits no marks of any mineral ſpirit. It is very ſlightly impregnated with *ſelenites*, and contains a ſmall portion of ſea ſalt. Some have ſuppoſed that it is a chalybeate, but without foundation.

20. THE Briſtol and Matlock waters appear to reſemble each other, both in their chemical and medicinal qualities.

21. MATLOCK bath raiſes Farenheit's thermometer to the 68th; the ſpring to the 66th. degree.

22. FIXED air may, in no inconſiderable quantity, be breathed without danger or uneaſineſs. And in ſeveral caſes of the *pthiſis pulmonalis*, the ſteams of an efferveſcing mixture of chalk and vinegar, have been inſpired with great advantage. Antiſeptic fumigations and vapours have been long employed and much extolled

extolled in ſuch diſorders. But their efficacy does not appear to depend on the extrication of fixed air from their ſubſtance.

23. THERE appears to be a diverſity in the properties and effects of different ſpecies of factitious air.

24. THE fixed air of metals ſeems to be of a kind different from that which is contained in alcalis and calcareous earth. And conſequently the action of theſe ſubſtances as *fluxes*, cannot be explained on the principle of their reſtoring the air, which had been loſt by calcination.

25. COMMON SALT, in the quantity of ten grains, promotes putrefaction; the *ſal catharticus amarus* in the ſame proportion is yet more ſeptic; but BAY SALT in this quantity reſiſts putrefaction; and GLAUBER'S SALT exceeds in this reſpect even bay ſalt. The ſeptic and antiſeptic qualities of theſe ſalts, when uſed in ſo minute

minute a quantity, are therefore evidently dependent on, and proportioned to their degrees of purity.

26. SEA SALT, and the bitter purging ſalt, though they quicken putrefaction, prevent the progreſs of it beyond a certain degree. A quality which muſt increaſe the uſefulneſs of the former, as a ſeaſoning to our food.

27. COFFEE is ſlightly aſtringent, and antiſeptic; moderates alimentary fermentation, and is powerfully ſedative. Its action on the nervous ſyſtem probably depends on the oil it contains; which receives its flavour, and is rendered mildly empyreumatic by the proceſs of roaſting.

SELECT

SELECT

HISTORIES OF DISEASES,

WITH

REMARKS.

Longum iter per precepta; breve et efficax per exempla.

SENECA.

* THE HISTORY AND CURE OF A DIFFICULTY IN DEGLUTITION OF LONG CONTINUANCE, ARISING FROM A SPASMODIC AFFECTION OF THE OESOPHAGUS.

MISS L—r, aged thirteen, a ſprightly girl, of a delicate and irritable habit of body, during ſeveral years had a difficulty of ſwallowing; which occaſionally left her for a month or two, and then ſuddenly returned without any apparent cauſe. September 3d, 1768, I was deſired to viſit her. She had then laboured under her diſorder ſix or eight months without any intermiſſion, and was reduced

* This Caſe was read before the College of Phyſicians, Auguſt 9, 1769, and is publiſhed in the Medical Tranſactions, Vol. 2.

duced almoſt to a ſkeleton, though ſhe ſtill retained her natural vivacity. When ſhe attempted to ſwallow ſolids, they paſſed down readily as far as the upper orifice of the ſtomach; but when arrived there, they were inſtantly, and with a ſtrong convulſive motion, thrown up again. Liquids ſipped ſlowly, and ſwallowed leiſurely, met with no reſiſtance; but when haſtily drunk, or in too large a quantity, they were quickly regurgitated. Warm liquors were ſwallowed with more eaſe than cold ones; and in the evening, the difficulty in deglutition generally abated. She complained of no other pain but an uneaſy craving in her ſtomach; nor was there any external ſwelling, or inward ſoreneſs, through the whole paſſage of the *œſophagus*. When ſhe was in her ninth year the *catamenia* appeared, and had recurred once or twice ſince that time, without any regularity. Her belly was coſtive, her pulſe was quick and ſmall, and her feet were uſu-

ally

ally cold. She was neither of a ſtrumous nor ſcorbutic habit of body; nor could her friends give me any ſatisfactory account of the origin or cauſe of her diſorder.

I APPREHENDED her caſe to be ſpaſmodic, complicated with a ſlight thickening of the *æſophagus* about the part affected, the conſequence of a contraction ſo long continued. The following medicines were therefore preſcribed.

℞. *Elixir. myrrhæ comp. tinct. valerian. vol. aa. ℨiv. M. dentur guttæ viginti in thea pulegii bis die.*

℞. *Ol. amygdal. ℥j. ſp. ſal. ammon. cum calce viva ℨvj. camphoræ oleo ſolutæ ℨij. ol. ſuccin. ℨiſs. M. f. linimentum, quo bene fricetur ſpina dorſi, a prima cervicis vertebra uſque ad duodeciman dorſalem, mane & veſperi quotidie.*

℞. *Merc.*

℞. *Merc. dulcis ſexies ſublimat. gr. ſs. mucilag. gum. Arab. ℈ij. ſp. nitri dulcis ℈ij. vin. antimon. gutt. vj. Aq. fontan. ℥ſs. Sacchari alb. ℈j. M. f. hauſt. hora decubitus quotidie ſumendus, vini antimonialis doſin ſenſim augendo.*

℞. *Extract. cort. Peruvian. mollis. caſtor. ruſſic. galban. colat. aa. partes æquales, camphoræ ſp. vin. rect. trit. ʒj. ol. ſuccini. ℈j. balſam. Peruvian. q. ſ. M. f. emplaſtrum ſcrobiculo cordis applicandum, & ſemel in ſeptimana renovandum.*

Directions were given that her feet and legs ſhould be kept warm; that her drinks ſhould not be taken cold; that her diet ſhould conſiſt of broth, mutton, or beef tea, as it is called, panada, vermicelli, ſago, rice, milk, chocolate, cocoa, ſalep, &c. that a little wine ſhould be occaſionally allowed;

ed; that ſhe ſhould abſtain from tea and coffee; that moderate exerciſe ſhould be daily uſed; and that a nouriſhing clyſter, prepared of milk, broth, &c. ſhould be injected every morning and noon; to obviate the looſening effect of which, a few red roſe leaves were ordered to be boiled in it, or a little ſtarch to be added to it.

September 22. THE liniment, calomel draught, and clyſter, had been neglected. But the plaſter had been applied; ſhe had taken the drops with regularity, and had carefully obſerved the regimen preſcribed to her. The difficulty in deglutition was ſenſibly abated, her appetite was mended, and ſhe had recovered fleſh and ſtrength.

October 1. THE mercurial draught had purged her. To prevent this effect, fifteen or twenty drops of *elixir paregoricum* were added. But a few days afterwards it occaſioned a ſoreneſs in her

 gums,

gums, and a ſlight ſalivation. The uſe of it was therefore diſcontinued.

October 21. SHE could now ſwallow ſolid food without any difficulty. Her appetite was good, her belly regular, her pulſe fuller and ſlower, her fleſh and ſtrength recruited, and her health in every other reſpect was perfectly re-eſtabliſhed. I directed her to continue the uſe of her medicines, and to perſevere in her regimen a month or two longer; and ſhe has ever ſince been entirely free from her diſorder.

I SHALL beg leave to make ſome general obſervations on obſtructed deglutition, without confining myſelf to the particular conſideration of the caſe which has been related.

1. A DIFFICULTY in ſwallowing may proceed from ſuch a variety of cauſes, not eaſy to be diſtinguiſhed, and yet each requiring

requiring a particular method of cure, that the phyſician's practice in ſuch caſes muſt be uncertain and perplexed. And what adds conſiderably to this embaraſſment is, that the effect often co-operates with the original cauſe, and confirms the diſeaſe. Thus a conſtriction of the *œſophagus*, ariſing from a ſpaſmodic affection, will, if it continue long, produce either an enlargement of the glands, or a thickening of the ſubſtance of the gullet, about the part affected. On the contrary, if the ſtricture proceed from a glandular tumour, from ſchirroſities, or fungous excreſcences, it will at the ſame time be complicated with ſome degree of ſpaſm; of which amongſt ſeveral inſtances that have fallen under my obſervation, I ſhall mention the following. A farmer's wife, aged fifty, of a ſtrumous habit, perceived an impediment in her throat to the paſſage of ſolid food, ſome months before ſhe applied for advice. Her diſorder had increaſed by degrees, and ſhe was then unable to ſwallow any thing but liquids. A ſurgeon examined the gullet with a probe, and found the two glands which are ſituated about the fifth vertebra of the back conſiderably enlarged. Æther was then a faſhionable remedy in this part of the country; and ſhe was induced, by the fame of its effects, to wiſh a trial might be made of it. A doſe properly diluted was given her, and about half an hour afterwards ſhe had the power of ſwallowing, without much difficulty, a morſel of ſolid food. But the relief was only temporary. She relapſed in an hour or two, and had again recourſe to the ſame remedy, which after a few trials loſt all its efficacy, and the poor woman having languiſhed about ſix months, died literally famiſhed. From this and other inſtances, I ſhould apprehend that the uſe of antiſpaſmodics would aſſiſt the operation of the mercurial courſe, ſo judiciouſly recommended by Doctor Munckley in the firſt volume of the Medical Tranſ-

actions;

actions; and would quicken, as well as render more certain, the cure of this deplorable diseafe.

2. In fpafmodic affections of the *æfophagus*, external applications to the fpine are likely to be very ferviceable, from the contiguity of that tube to the *vertebræ*. And perhaps nothing would be more effectual in fuch cafes than a blifter, applied either to the neck or between the fhoulders. That epifpaftics are powerful antifpafmodics, experience hath fully afcertained; and where the diforder is attended with an enlargement of the fubftance, or a fullnefs of the glands of the gullet, they would have additional efficacy, by producing a copious difcharge of ferous humours, and by that means unloading the veffels of the part affected.

Volatile and antifpafmodic liniments are alfo highly ufeful, as the cafe above recited fufficiently evinces. It is indeed to be lamented that external applications of this kind are not more frequently employed in practice; for there is just reason to apprehend that powerful effects might be expected from them in various diseases. In the hooping cough particularly, I have observed considerable benefit to accrue from the use of a liniment, similar to the one prescribed above.

3. When constrictions of the *œsophagus,* arising from spasm, have been of long continuance, and do not yield to medicine; electricity furnishes us with no improbable means of relief. The publick indeed have been much disappointed in the medical effects of electricity. But this hath in part proceeded from the misapplication of so powerful a remedy. It appears to me, and I am confirmed in this opinion by the observation of a very eminent physician, that the electric shock bids fair to do much more good in

in diseases from rigidity, than in those from laxity. Amongst many other proofs of this, may be adduced the cure of a universal *tetanus*, the history of which is published by Doctor Watson, in one of the late volumes of the Philosophical Transactions.

4. STIMULATING vapours conveyed into the *pharynx* have a tendency to remove spasms, even when seated deep in the *œsophagus*. A few years ago an elderly gentlewoman, after eating pease, felt an uneasy sensation as if one of them stuck low down in her throat, and suddenly found herself deprived of the power of deglutition. Notwithstanding the use of a variety of remedies, her inability to swallow continued five or six days. She was directed to fumigate her throat with *assafœtida*, dissolved in a strong infusion of the aromatic herbs: and drawing in the vapours very forcibly, the spasm was in-

ſtantly reſolved; nor has ſhe ever ſince ſuffered the leaſt return of it.

5. When this dreadful diſeaſe is ſo confirmed as to be deemed incurable, the patient's life may be prolonged by the daily injection of nutritive clyſters, and by bathing his feet, hands, and arms, and occaſionally his whole body, in new milk, broth, decoctions of ſalep, ſago, or vermicelli, &c. The abſorption by the lymphatics of the ſkin is very conſiderable. It has been found by experiment that the hand, after being well chafed, will imbibe in a quarter of an hour near an ounce and a half of warm water. And allowing that the ſurface of the hand is to that of the body as one to ſixty, the abſorption of the whole, in the ſame ſpace of time, would amount to upwards of ſeven pounds. The copious diſcharge of urine in the *diabetes*, ſo much exceeding in quantity the patient's drink, confirms

in

in ſome meaſure this calculation. And the curious fact related by Dr. Chalmers, at the ſame time that it affords a further proof of the great abſorption by the pores of the ſkin, points out to us the valuable purpoſes to which it may be applied in the diſorder under conſideration. A negro man, who had eaten or drunk but little before he was gibbetted in March, 1759, at Charles Town in South Carolina, and had nothing given him afterwards, regularly voided every morning a large quantity of urine, but diſcharged no more till about the ſame hour the next day. The dews of the evening, imbibed by the body, ſupplied in this caſe a ſuperabundance of fluids in the night, and a ſufficient quantity to ſupport perſpiration in the day. Had theſe fluids been of a nutritious quality, it is not improbable that, even under ſuch circumſtances, the poor negro might have been kept alive for a conſiderable length of time.

PROSPER

Prosper Alpinus relates that the Egyptian women, in order to become fat, uſe every day a tepid bath; and whilſt they continue in it, receive nouriſhing clyſters, and a variety of the richeſt foods. By this means the females of that country, particularly the Hebrew women who reſide there, are for the moſt part immoderately corpulent. *Illarum plurimæ perinde ac ſues cernuntur pinguiſſimæ humi recumbentes, maximeque Hebreæ, quibus iſtud vitii aliis familiarius obſervatur.*

I have not enlarged upon the neceſſity of conveying aliment into the body by clyſters, in obſtructions of the *æſophagus*, becauſe this muſt be obvious to every practitioner. The other method of nutrition, if not leſs known, is certainly leſs attended to, and in general is altogether neglected. It may perhaps be thought an omiſſion, that no notice has been taken of the adminiſtration of medicines

cines under the form of clyſters, in theſe deplorable caſes. But I apprehend, however uſeful they might be in many reſpects, they would in general too much interfere with the nouriſhment of the patient.

CASES

OF

DROPSIES.

CASE I.

MRS. POPPLETON, aged 33, a woman of a very delicate conſtitution, and ſubject to a *profluvium menſium*, which had greatly impaired her ſtrength, perceived about two years ago an indolent, moveable tumour in the lower part and left ſide of her belly, which gradually though ſlowly increaſed. Before it acquired any conſiderable bulk, her right leg began to ſwell, her urine was voided in in ſmall quantity; the ſymptoms of thirſt and inward heat enſued; the *abdomen* became enlarged; a fluctuation was ſoon perceptible; and a complete *aſcites* was formed.

THE tumour in the lower part of her belly, which from its ſituation I apprehend was an incyſted dropſy of the left *ovarium,* now began to be extremely painful, the ſwelling of the *abdomen* increaſed, a general *anaſarca* was coming on, and her caſe became every day more and more deplorable. Things were in this ſtate, when the patient, as ſhe aroſe out of bed in the morning (February 2d, 1771,) was ſeized with a nauſea, without any apparent cauſe, which was ſoon ſucceeded by a violent vomiting. At three o'clock in the afternoon I was firſt called to her aſſiſtance, and found her quite exhauſted with inceſſant reachings. Her pulſe was ſo feeble as to be ſcarcely perceptible, her extremities were cold, and her legs and thighs were affected with a moſt painful ſpaſm. She had diſcharged near ten pints of water, and this evacuation had entirely removed the anaſarcous ſwellings, and greatly diminiſhed the fullneſs and tenſion of the belly. The tumour of the left *ovarium,* though much decreaſed in bulk, was evident to the touch, and appeared to be ſtill moveable under the fingers. Gentle cordials were directed to ſupport the patient's ſtrength, warm fomentations were applied to her legs and thighs, and an opiate was adminiſtered, to procure for her a ſhort interval of reſt and eaſe. She enjoyed a few hours refreſhing ſleep; the vomiting then recurred, and continued five or ſix days, with intermiſſions, which gradually became longer and longer. Her thirſt during theſe evacuations was almoſt inſupportable, but ſhe refrained with great reſolution from all liquids, except a little red port wine diluted with mint water. O-

ranges

ranges too were freely allowed, and were highly grateful to her. All her dropſical ſwellings were now removed, and the tumour of the *ovarium* itſelf was no longer perceptible. When the vomiting ceaſed, a gentle *diarrhœa* ſucceeded. An infuſion of the bark with the *ſp. nitr. dulcis.* and *tinct. mart. in ſp. ſalis* were given. Her thirſt abated, her appetite returned, and in a few weeks ſhe recovered a tolerable degree of health and ſtrength, and ſtill continues free from any of her former ailments, though it is now four months from the time when her vomitings commenced. The quantity of water ſhe diſcharged, excluſive of her evacuations by ſtool and urine, amounted to about three gallons.

THE caſe before us affords a ſtriking proof of the efforts which nature exerts to relieve herſelf. By what ſecret inſtruments this ſalutary change was produced in the preſent inſtance, we may conjecture,

ture, but cannot aſcertain. It is not to be ſuppoſed that the extravaſated fluids paſſed by percolation through the coats of the ſtomach or inteſtines, and were then diſcharged by vomiting; becauſe theſe coats in the living body are impervious to water, and tranſmit it only when the circulation ceaſes, when their veſſels ſhrink, and the *mucus* lining the internal cavity is dried or abraded. Nor is it eaſy to conceive, how the hydropic cyſt of the *ovarium* ſhould thus empty itſelf into the ventricle; or ſo large a quantity of water tranſude with ſuch rapidity, through the interſtices of its fibres. For that the ſtomach was not ruptured is evident from the ſpeedy recovery of the patient. The effect therefore muſt be aſcribed, not to a mechanical cauſe, but to that vital energy which by imperceptible means regulates the motions, and corrects the diſorders of the animal frame; though ſometimes with a degree of violence dangerous to, and even deſtructive of life. In the preſent

present caſe it appears probable, that a ſudden change took place in the courſe of circulation; the lymphatics recovered their power of abſorption, and performed their office with renewed vigour; the vaſcular ſyſtem became overloaded, and the exhalant arteries of the ſtomach and inteſtines poured forth the ſuperfluous fluids, reſtoring thus the equilibrium.

INSTANCES of a ſudden, and partially increaſed action of the veſſels frequently occur, as in the *diarrhœa, cholera morbus,* hyſteric diſeaſe, *profluvium urinæ,* &c. &c. But the following hiſtory, related by Doctor Simſon, admirably illuſtrates, and at the ſame time confirms what I have advanced. *Cum homo adoleſcens, febri correptus, cui aceſſerat diarrhœa, cum extremo ſtupore ſenſuum, nihil plane ore haurire vellet, (quamquam immoderato æſtu totus torreſceret) quo humectaretur, jubeo in aquam egelidam imergi pedes; quo facto, protinus aquæ mirum cerno in vaſe decrementum,*

 deinde

deinde ejuſdem vixdum coloratæ, e veſtigio impetuoſam, more cataractæ, per anum effuſionem. (*a*)

SEVERAL inſtances are recorded of anaſarcas, and ſome few even of the aſcites, which have been cured by vomiting. But I believe it has rarely if ever happened, at leaſt I do not recollect ſuch a caſe either in books or in practice, that a dropſy of the *ovarium* has been removed by the ſpontaneous efforts of nature. Deductions from ſingular and ſolitary facts, though contrary to the rules of philoſophiſing, are not always to be rejected; but may be allowed with proper caution and reſerve, when the nature of the ſubject admits not of better evidence. The hiſtory before us furniſhes, I apprehend, an exception to the general laws of reaſoning by induction; and one inſtance, well authenticated, of the cure of

(*a*) Simſon de Re Medica, p. 183.

of a diſeaſe, which the moſt eminent phyſicians have conſidered as irremediable, may juſtly lead us, in ſimilar circumſtances, to imitate by art the operations of nature; and to excite thoſe efforts, which when ſpontaneous, have proved ſo ſalutary. In the incipient ſtate of a dropſy of the *ovarium*, emetics repeatedly adminiſtered would be likely means of promoting the abſorption or diſcharge of the incyſted fluid. They produce the ſtrongeſt contractions in the abdominal muſcles, agitate all the viſcera of the lower belly, quicken the circulation of the blood, and by their general action on the whole ſyſtem, remove obſtructions in the minuteſt and moſt remote ſeries of veſſels. Hence the powerful effects of Turpeth vomits in white ſwellings of the joints; in which the glands are at leaſt equally diſeaſed, and the extravaſated fluid as much out of the courſe of the circulation, as in the ſpecies of dropſy we are now conſidering. But unfortunately this diſorder is ſo inſidious in its attack, and ſo little alarming in its progreſs, that it becomes almoſt incurable before the patient is apprehenſive of any degree of danger. However in its more advanced ſtages, emetics may be adminiſtered with ſafety, and ſometimes perhaps with advantage. If the *morſus diaboli* adhere to the enlarged *ovarium*, and the fallopian tubes be not totally obſtructed, the action of vomiting may force a paſſage for the fluid, and thus procure at leaſt ſome temporary relief. I have now under my care a lady who has long been afflicted with a dropſy of this kind, and who has frequent diſcharges of bloody water from the womb, ſucceeded always by a diminution of bulk. A troubleſome *hernia* forbids the exhibition of an emetic, which otherwiſe I ſhould not heſitate to direct. Beſides we may poſſibly be ſo fortunate as to co-operate with nature at the moſt favourable conjuncture, and by aſſiſting her efforts, of themſelves perhaps too

too languid, may effect a cure. Such inſtances do not unfrequently occur, in almoſt every ſpecies of diſeaſe; and it is upon this principle alone, that we can explain the amazing ſucceſs which has attended the exhibition of remedies, by no means adequate to the effects produced by them. Mr. W. a hard drinker, when paſt the meridian of life, had a jaundice which was ſucceeded by an *aſcites*, a dropſy of the *thorax*, and an *anaſarca*. The prognoſtic was in this caſe extremely unfavourable, and I ſcarcely indulged the leaſt hope of his recovery. Diuretics, purgatives, &c. under various forms, were aſſiduouſly adminiſtered, but with no very advantageous effects. Amongſt other medicines he took pills compoſed of *extract. jalap. pulv. ſcillar. ſiccat.* and *merc. dulcis.* and was directed to increaſe the doſe of theſe *pro re nata*. Finding the uſual quantity inſufficient to procure the neceſſary diſcharges, he took, if I recollect

collect aright, two pills extraordinary, the consequence of which was an *hypercatharsis*, which greatly reduced his strength, but carried off all his dropsical swellings, and by the aid of cordials and corroborants, produced a perfect cure. The following curious case, communicated to me by a physician of eminence in a neighbouring town, further illustrates the observation advanced above; and at the same time shews the resources which medicine affords to a sagacious practitioner, in the most desperate stages of this disorder.

CASE II.

Miss H. of Namptwich in Cheshire, aged upwards of forty, had laboured for some time under an *ascites*, when she was removed to Liverpool in February 1769, for the benefit of medical advice. Two physicians and a surgeon were consulted, and after a gentle evacuation by ſtool, and the exhibition of a few cardiacs, it was agreed that ſhe ſhould be tapped without delay. Eighteen pints of water were drawn off, and two large ſchirrous tumours, one nearly the ſize of an infant's head, the other not much leſs in bulk, were diſcovered. Theſe ſhe had perceived for many years, and they had ſucceeded a fever, imperfect in its criſis. The operation had almoſt proved fatal to her; her mouth was covered with *aphthæ*, and ſo many alaıming ſymptoms came on, that death was hourly expected. However in a fortnight ſhe was tolerably recovered, and in a month the *paracenteſis* was again repeated. She bore it better, but ſoon filled again, and was obliged to ſubmit to the operation every third week. Tired with the frequency of this painful palliative, after the fifteenth repetition of it, ſhe requeſted one of her phyſicians in a moſt preſſing manner, to preſcribe ſome medicine, which might at leaſt protract

M 4 the

the period of tapping. It was now the latter end of Auguſt, the weather was favourable, and he directed her to be confined to her bed for three days, to be aſſiduouſly rubbed morning and evening with dry cloths impregnated with the fumes of camphor, and to take internally the *julepum e camphora*, prepared with only two-thirds of a pint of water, and warmed with the addition of one ounce of *aqua juniperi compoſita*. Under this form ſhe took a drachm of camphor daily, for the ſpace of a fortnight. A continued gentle *diaphoreſis* was the happy conſequence; every day ſhe decreaſed in bulk, and the abatement of her ſwellings encouraged her reſolutely to perſevere in the uſe of her medicine. She recovered her health, and remained near two years free from any dropſical complaints. But in the ſummer of 1771, her diſorder recurred; and on the 16th. of July ſhe was again tapped. On the 8th. of October following, ſhe voided by the *anus* near twelve pints

pints of a mucilaginous liquor, in colour reſembling *pus*, but without any offenſive ſmell. After this remarkable diſcharge, ſhe was better for a ſhort time; but a violent and very painful aphthous complaint, attended with a profuſe ſpitting of viſcid phlegm and ſaliva, then enſued; by which her ſtrength was exhauſted, and ſhe died on the 9th. of November, quite emaciated.

On the ſame day her body was opened in the preſence of two phyſicians, and other gentlemen of the faculty; and I am favoured by Mr. Wickſted, a very ingenious ſurgeon at Namptwich, who attended the patient during her laſt illneſs, with the following account of the appearances on diſſection.

"On opening the abdomen a large hard tumour preſented itſelf, which on examination, ſeemed to be the right *ova-*

ovarium very much enlarged, and ſchirrous. It was in figure like an impregnated *uterus*, filling the lower ſpace of the abdomen, and riſing ſeveral inches above the brim of the *pelvis*. This ſubſtance, was found attached to the *uterus*, and weighed three pounds and ſeven ounces. By its preſſure the *uterus* and bladder were forced down into the lower part of the *pelvis*; and when divided, it reſembled a piece of boiled udder in colour and firmneſs.

The left *ovarium* was very hard, and enlarged to the ſize of a gooſe egg. The body of the *uterus*, which with the bladder had been preſſed by the weight of the tumour out of its uſual ſituation, was hardly to be diſtinguiſhed from the left *ovarium*, which was nearly of the ſame ſize and firmly united with it, and ſeemed to be a little diſeaſed. The fallopian tubes were almoſt obliterated. The bladder and ureters were ſound.

The

The hydropic cyſt, (which extended to the margin of the ribs, and appeared to be formed either from the diſtended peritonæal coats of the *ovaria*, or the duplicatures of the *peritonæum)* contained three quarters of a pint of a fluid, ſimilar to that which had been evacuated by ſtool.

The ſtomach and inteſtines were in a ſound ſtate, and no where adhered to the above-mentioned cyſt. But at the bottom of the *pelvis* the cyſt had a *firm attachment to the rectum* of the compaſs of half a crown; yet there was no viſible perforation, by which ſo large a quantity of fluids could eſcape. The omentum was waſted to a membranous expanſion. The kidnies, ſpleen, pancreas, and meſenteric glands were ſound. The ſubſtance of the liver was not at all diſeaſed, but its whole convex ſurface was fixed by ſtrong adheſions to the *diaphragm*. Both lobes of the lungs were found adhering to the *pleura*; their internal ſtructure however ſeemed

ſeemed to be perfect. The heart was in a good ſtate; and the *pericardium* contained about two ounces of limpid water."

CASE III.

Mr. G. H. of Oldham, near Mancheſter, aged upwards of fifty, low of ſtature, corpulent, and habitually addicted to intemperance, in April, 1770, was afflicted with a dry cough, *dyſpnæa*, *aſcites*, and ſwelled legs. By the uſe of pills compoſed of *ſapo venet. gum. ammoniac.* and *pulv. ſcillar.* and a ſmart mercurial cathartic, which I directed to be repeated at ſuch intervals as not to debilitate his ſtrength, he recovered his former ſtate of health. But on the 2d. of January, 1771, I was again called to his aſſiſtance; he had been ſuddenly ſeized a few days before with a difficulty of breathing, which increaſed faſt, and was then attended with a cough and frothy expectoration; his pulſe

pulſe was languid and oppreſſed, his heat natural, his face bloated, and his legs were ſlightly œdematous; the *abdomen* was not fuller than uſual, nor had he previous to his attack, any ſymptoms of water in the cavity of the cheſt. A briſk purgative, *radix Senekæ*, *oxymel ſcillit.* bliſters to the legs, *camphor*, *ſal. volatile*, *venæſection*, &c. &c. were tried, but without effect. Reſpiration became more and more laborious, and in two days the patient was freed from his ſufferings by death.

IT appears probable to me that an *anaſarca*, or infarction of the cellular membrane of the lungs, was the proximate cauſe of the *orthopnœa*, which in ſo ſhort a time proved fatal to the unhappy patient. This diſorder may, like other dropſies, ariſe from a general laxity of the ſolids, tenuity of the fluids, or obſtructed circulation of the blood; but in ſuch inſtances it will in all probability be ſlowly

and

and gradually produced. How then are we to account for its ſudden and rapid formation in the caſe I have juſt related? The ancient phyſicians who had no opportunities of diſſecting human bodies, obſerved in brutes, particularly in oxen, ſheep, and ſwine, large hydatids in the lungs; and to the rupture of theſe, Hippocrates and Galen, reaſoning from analogy, aſcribed the *hydrops pectoris* in the human ſpecies. Willis and Morgagni have adopted their opinion, and confirmed the teſtimony of the father of phyſic, and his learned commentators. Morgagni ſays, *In ſue autem, cæteroquin ſano, ut cætera ejuſmodi hic omittam, a me in beſtiis, hominibuſque conſpecta, hydatidem vidiſſe memini, quæ minorem ſui partem in pulmonis ſuperficie oſtendens, interius adeo ſe amplificabat, ut aquæ limpidæ uncias aliquot contineret.* (a) And another laborious anatomiſt

(a) Morgagni de cauſis & ſedibus Morb. Epiſt. 16. Art. 36.

tomiſt (*Bonetus in Sepulch. Anatom. Obſ.* 33 and 36,) informs us that the lungs of a man were found full of bladders, which when opened, diſcharged either water, or a clear liquor reſembling the white of an egg. Theſe obſervations I think point out the cauſe, and at the ſame time account for the rapid progreſs and fatal termination of the pulmonary *œdema*, under which my patient laboured. Some hydatids, contained in the cellular membrane of the lungs, were probably ruptured internally, and in an habit abounding with the *colluvies ſeroſa*, the extravaſated fluids would be every inſtant accumulating, and the bronchial veſicles, becoming more and more compreſſed, ſuffocation inevitably enſued.

THE diagnoſtics of the *hydrops pectoris*, whether the water be contained in the cellular membrance of the lungs, or in the cavity of the cheſt, are ſometimes very obſcure. Doctor Hoadly relates that he was

was preſent at the diſſection of a dropſical man, from the ſymptoms of whoſe diſeaſe it was with ſuch certainty concluded, that water was contained in one ſide of the breaſt, that the only motive for examination was to determine into which cavity the fluid was extravaſated. On opening his body however they diſcovered not a ſingle drop of water, but found an almoſt total adheſion of the external coat of the lungs to the pleura; together with an inflammation, and numberleſs ſmall ulcers in one lobe.

A SENSIBLE fluctuation of water in the breaſt is a ſymptom which rarely occurs, and it appears from Morgagni's obſervations, that it is not unuſual for patients labouring under this diſorder, to bear with eaſe a recumbent poſture. But an *œdema* or dropſy of the cellular membrance of the lungs, when its attack is ſudden, may often be diſtinguiſhed by the following ſigns, although it muſt be acknowledged

knowledged that they ſometimes prove equivocal. The difficulty in reſpiration is conſtant, and increaſed by the leaſt motion, though not much varied by different attitudes of the body; the patient complains of great anxiety about the *præcordia*, and when he attempts to take a deep inſpiration, he finds it impoſſible to dilate his cheſt, and his breath ſeems to be ſuddenly ſtopped. The pulſe is ſmall, languid, and oppreſſed; the face pale and bloated; the legs uſually ſwelled, and the whole habit is for the moſt part leucophlegmatic.

A DISEASE ſo urgent in its ſymptoms, ſo quick in its progreſs, and ſo often fatal in its termination, requires a method of cure of adequate expedition and efficacy. A briſk mercurial cathartic, which will not only unload the internal canal, but promote abſorption, by ſtimulating and increaſing the action of the whole vaſcular ſyſtem, ſhould be adminiſtered without delay. I have lately ſeen ſurpriſing relief in a very alarming caſe, almoſt inſtantly procured by ſuch a remedy. (a) Bliſters to the legs have alſo ſometimes a good effect; for by deſtroying the cuticle, and *rete mucoſum*, they diſcharge the water from the cellular membrane of a depending part, and thus in ſome degree produce a general depletion. Punctures made with a ſmall lancet, or with ſuch an inſtrument as Doctor Fothergill has lately recommended, will anſwer the ſame end; and be leſs liable to produce pain and inflammation. Diuretics, ſudorifics, and expectorants, as they all increaſe the more fluid excretions, are indicated in this diſeaſe. And if the moſt powerful medicines of one claſs fail, recourſe ſhould immediately be had to another. Seneka root in liberal doſes ſometimes anſwers every intention, and operates powerfully by the ſkin, the kidneys, and the

(a) A ſimilar caſe is recorded by Dr. Simſon, in the Edin. Med. Eſſays, Vol. 6. p. 126.

the bronchial glands, to the great relief of the patient. But if the moſt active medicines prove ineffectual, and the aggravation of all the ſymptoms threaten almoſt inſtant diſſolution, might not the *paracenteſis* of the lungs be attempted with ſafety, and advantage? *Melius eſt anceps remedium quam nullum*, is an eſtabliſhed maxim in phyſic, and certainly in this inſtance would juſtify the trial of an operation which is neither very painful, nor likely to be attended with any dangerous conſequences. Many caſes have been recorded of wounds in the lungs, which have been healed, without much difficulty. Nor have ſuch accidents been ſucceeded by an *emphyſema*; for it may be concluded from Mr. Hewſon's ingenious experiments that a puncture or inciſion will not occaſion any emiſſion of air, into the cavity of the *thorax*, on account of the effuſion of blood, and ſubſequent inflammation, by which the divided veſicles are firſt filled, and afterwards entirely cloſed.

closed. To produce a discharge of air, a laceration or superficial abrasion of the lungs seems to be necessary; and hence it is that fractured ribs are the most frequent causes of the *emphysema*.

SHOULD the *paracentesis* of the lungs ever be deemed expedient, the chest may be perforated by cautiously dissecting with a knife, as in the operation for the *empyema*. If the lungs adhere to the *pleura* where the incision is made, they may be punctured with a lancet, and the water will thus be discharged without falling into the cavity of the *thorax*; but a trocar will be necessary to obviate as much as possible this inconvenience, if there be no adhesion. The operation, for evident reasons, should first be performed on the right side, and if this do not afford the patient sufficient relief, another opening may be made between the seventh and eighth ribs of the left side, in order to avoid the *pericardium*.

CASE

CASE OF A PALSY, ARISING FROM THE EFFLUVIA OF LEAD, IN WHICH ELECTRICITY WAS SUCCESSFULLY EMPLOYED.

ELECTRICITY, like all other active remedies, may prove injurious as well as beneficial to the human body, and it is to be regretted that experience has not yet ſupplied us with any certain *criteria*, by which to determine when it will be hurtful, when innocent, or efficacious. That analogy may deceive us is evident from many examples. A girl, about ſixteen, who had loſt the uſe of her arm, which was greatly waſted, became univerſally paralytic, after being electrified; and remained ſo above a fortnight.

night. The general palſy was removed by proper medicines; but the diſeaſed arm continued as before. Electricity was again tried, and repeated three or four days, when the girl became a ſecond time univerſally paralytic, and even loſt the uſe of her tongue. By a courſe of medicine ſhe was once more relieved from this additional palſy; but the original one, which affected her arm, remained incurable. *(a)* A gentleman, aged forty-eight, inclined to corpulency, and of a phlegmatic temperament, had a paralytic affection of the leg and thigh. Electricity was tried, but the ſlighteſt ſhocks always increaſed the torpor of the limb. The ſame gentleman, twelve months afterwards, was attacked with an *hemiplegia*. To gratify his inclination, and contrary to my own judgement, I conſented to the uſe of electricity a ſecond time: and this remedy, which had before proved

(a) Vid. Philoſ. Tranſact. Vol. 48, p. 786; alſo, Prieſtley's Hiſtory of Electricity, p. 386.

proved injurious, was now at leaſt innocent, and even thought to be beneficial to him.

THE electrical ſhock incautiouſly communicated, may be productive of dangerous and even fatal conſequences. Mr. R. aged fifty, ſubject to various nervous and hypochondriacal complaints, after ſuffering ſeveral ſlight paralytic affections, which yielded to medicine, was at length deprived of the uſe of one ſide. Electricity, and other active remedies, were applied. Gentle ſhocks were repeatedly given by a ſkilful perſon; and the patient ſeemed to receive benefit from each operation. But by an unfortunate miſtake in the poſition of the chain, the ſhock was one day conveyed through the epigaſtric region, and not along the paralytic arm, which reſted upon it. A violent pain was inſtantly perceived in the ſtomach, which in a few minutes was ſucceeded by a profuſe vomiting of blood. The hæmorrhage continued two or three days, and ſo exhauſted the ſtrength of the patient, as certainly to accelerate, and perhaps to occaſion his death.

PALSIES frequently ſucceed the *colica pictonum*, whether owing to ſome nervous ſympathy between the bowels and the limbs, or to the tranſlation of any morbid acrimony, cannot eaſily be determined. In ſuch caſes, the waters of Bath in Somerſetſhire are highly beneficial; and electricity, it is probable, would be a uſeful auxiliary to them. When the circumſtances of the patient render a journey to thoſe celebrated ſprings impracticable or inconvenient, the latter remedy may be tried alone with ſome proſpect of ſucceſs. Of this the following curious caſe, communicated to me by Dr. Withering, affords a preſumptive proof.

"JOSEPH

" JOSEPH ADAMS, aged 20, was admitted into the Stafford infirmary on the 16th. of September, 1768. Some months ago he felt a numbneſs and coldneſs in the left leg and thigh, which gradually extended all over him, his head excepted, which is now the only part he can move. His limbs are often ſeized with involuntary twitchings, as in the *chorea ſ. vitæ.* Pulſe natural. Appetite good. Coſtive. This man was formerly uſed to work in lead mines, at which time he was often ſenſible of a ſweet taſte in his mouth; but for two years paſt has been employed in digging a navigable canal, and has been much expoſed to wet and cold. An antimonial vomit, a mercurial purge, and an emulſion, with a large proportion of *ol. olivar.* were preſcribed.

ON the 21ſt. He could move his right arm, and his legs a little, as he lay in bed. A number of ſmall electrical ſhocks

ſhocks were paſſed through both arms, and ordered to be repeated daily.

23d. SWEATS after being electrified; is univerſally warmer; can ſtir his left arm.

24th. FEELS a tingling in his right arm. His fingers contract upon the chain, when the ſhock paſſes. The frequency of his pulſe is not increaſed during the operation. Electrify all his limbs.

27th. CAN ſhut both his hands, and bring the right up to his mouth, when lying in bed; but not when raiſed up.

29th. FEELS the ſhocks more ſenſibly than he did at firſt. They always excite a ſtrong tingling ſenſation. When raiſed upon his feet, can ſtand upright betwixt two aſſiſtants.

AT this time it was diſcovered that he had ſeveral venereal ſhankers, and an ulcer

cer upon the *glans penis*. The electricity was discontinued, and a course of sublimate solution, and mercurial unction entered upon; by which means all the venereal symptoms were subdued.

November 30th. His paralytic complaints being just in the same state as on the 29th. of September, recourse was again had to the electrical machine; and two large spoonfuls of *ol. olivar.* were given twice a day, to prevent costiveness.

December 18th. Sweats when electrified: has more motion in his body; feeds himself in bed, but cannot when up. The fingers sometimes drawn inwards, so as almost to touch the palms of his hands; his arms and legs always benumbed, except for a short time after the use of the machine.

28th. Palsy much the same; for the relief gained at the time of electrifying

ing ceaſes in a ſhort time after it is over. Continues very coſtive. The antimonial vomit was repeated; a drachm of *pilul. gummos.* ordered to be taken twice in a day, with three ounces of the decoction of Peruvian bark. Omit the electricity.

January 10th, 1769. THESE medicines at firſt gave him ſtools, but they have not now that effect. The palſy in the ſame ſtate. Complains of great pain in the right ſhoulder, and right ſide of the neck. A bliſter was applied to the neck, the pills continued, and the bark decoction changed for four ounces of paralytic infuſion. An ounce of volatile liniment was ordered to be rubbed daily upon the ſpine; iſſues to be made in the thighs; and when the bliſter healed, a ſeton in his neck. He continued nearly in this method until the 12th. of April, without any other advantage than being free from his pains. He was ordered into

into the warm bath, every other day, and to take as much of the freſh leaves of cuckow pint * twice every day, as his ſtomach would bear.

May 3d. THE cuckow pint creates an uncommon heat in his ſtomach, but produces no other ſenſible effect. Let bliſters be applied to his legs, and afterwards to the lower part of the ſpine.

28th. THE palſy continuing in the ſame ſtate, recourſe was again had to electricity.

Auguſt 21ſt. HAS improved, though very ſlowly, in ſtrength and motion. The muſcles of his back allow him to ſtoop, and raiſe himſelf again: the right arm nearly as ſtrong as when in health; but for more than a week paſt his palſy has continued the ſame, and he complains of griping

* Arum Maculatum, *Linnæi* Species Plantarum.

griping pains in his belly, which is tenſe and very coſtive. The uſual medicines not giving him ſtools, let him take a large ſpoonful of caſtor oil every morning. Continue the electricity.

September 6th. FREE from the pain in his belly; the caſtor oil purges him conſiderably. Has more uſe in his left arm, and ſweats profuſely after electrifying.

13th. STOOD himſelf to day.

November 10th. CAN raiſe himſelf from his chair, and ſtand without help.

22d. WALKS about, with the aſſiſtance of his chair.

December 17th. DURING this month was a good deal afflicted with the gravel, which gave way to the uſual remedies.

27th. WALKS with one ſtick.

January

January 3d, 1770. BEGINS to walk without a ſtick. From this time he continued mending until the 11th. of May; when he was diſcharged perfectly cured.

THE firſt circumſtance that ſtrikes our attention in the hiſtory of this diſeaſe is the diſtance of time betwixt the patient's expoſure to the deleterious *effluvia* of the lead mines, and the appearance of the palſy. That the palſy was occaſioned by lead is moſt probable; as there ſeemed to be through the whole of the cure, more or leſs of the *colica pictonum* exiſting. The effects of the caſtor oil in this diſeaſe are too evident to paſs unnoticed; eſpecially as I have heard ſome very ingenious and candid practitioners aſſert, that they have found no more purgative quality in that oil, than in an equal quantity of olive oil. The medicine they uſed muſt have been highly adulterated.

THAT electricity does not afford relief in

in paralytic complaints, after five days application, has been aſſerted by a very ingenious philoſopher; and I am afraid it is an opinion which has been too generally received. Dr. De Haen in his *Ratio Medendi* produces inſtances to the contrary; but none more ſtriking than the above caſe, wherein it appears that the palſy continued in the ſame ſtate, whenever the ſhocks were omitted. Patients are frequently diſcouraged by the painful ſenſation which large ſhocks excite, from perſevering in an electrical courſe; and it is not uncommon to find, that any given degree of ſhock will occaſion more pain in a diſeaſed, and even in a paralytic limb, than in a ſound one: I cannot omit adding, that I have never met with a caſe which reſiſted the power of ſmall and repeated ſhocks, that would yield to great and terrifying ſtrokes. Like other active and uſeful remedies, electricity may be given in too large a doſe, and may then produce conſiderable miſchief.

mifchief. Nor are there wanting feveral well authenticated facts, to fupport this opinion. The largeft fhock I have ever found ufeful, has been from an eight ounce phial, coated in the common manner; and even this in many irritable habits, is confiderably too ftrong. For there is an amazing difference in the fenfibility of different conftitutions to the electrical ftimulus. Quick, lively people feel the moft from it; thofe the leaft, who are dull and flow of apprehenfion.

CASES

OF

OBSTINATE CHOLICS,

CURED BY

THE USE OF ALUM.

A DUTCH writer of confiderable merit, but not generally known in England, has recommended the ufe of alum in the *colica pictonum*, and in other obftinate and painful affections of the bowels, and has favoured the public with feveral well authenticated hiftories of its beneficial effects. *(a)*

I HAVE

(a) DE Colica Pictonum Tentamen, & Appendix, auctore, Joanne Grafhuis, M.D.

" CURA-

I HAVE adminiſtered this remedy in about fifteen caſes; with a degree of ſucceſs which confirms his teſtimony, and induces me to propoſe it to the trial of other phyſicians. The doſe in which I have given it, has uſually been, from ten to twenty

"CURATIONIS methodus (colicæ ſcilicet pictonum) quatuor indicationibus abſolvitur. Expoſtulat 1. lenimen doloris, nulla habita ad cauſam ſpecialem ratione. 2. Cauſæ proximæ vel ablationem vel extinctionem. 3. Partium affectarum in integram, quantum fieri poſſit, reſtitutionem. 4. Alvi interea temporis, difficillime in pleriſque conſtipatæ, toto curationis decurſu exſolutionem. Prima indicatio anodyna expoſcit; ſecunda demulcentia; tertia roborantia. Sine his, levatio morbi duabus prioribus indicationibus impetrata, raro tuta fidaque eſt, hiſce ſolis aliquando curatio integre abſolvitur abſque ùllo aliorum extradictis jam indicationibus præſidio. Siquidem haud raro vidi morbum anodynis & demulcentibus, ſeorſum et per ſe, vel combinatis; ſat magna copia & ſatis diu aſſumptis, vinci non potuiſſe: in quibus caſibus omni ſpe ſanationis impetrandæ abjecta, roborantibus fortioribus non calidis, ut inteſtinorum tonus relaxatus emendaretur, adhibitis, invincibilem ut videbatur hoſtem profligari feliciter. Quare hæc methodus a me tentata, deinceps mihi maxime commendabilis fuit; eoque felicior quo medicamentorum adſtrictoria potentia major, eorumque propinatio liber alior diuturniorque."

De Colica Pictonum, p. 48.

twenty grains, mixed with an equal proportion of ſugar. When there was reaſon to apprehend that it might be too rough and auſtere in its action, I have directed it to be combined with gum arabic or *ſperma ceti:* and in caſes of flatulence, when a warm opiate was indicated, half a ſcruple of the *philonium Londinenſe,* made a uſeful addition to it. Fifteen grains of alum given every fourth, fifth, or ſixth hour, for the moſt part prove gently aperient; and when the ſymptoms are not very ſevere, the ſecond or third doſe ſeldom fails to mitigate the pain, and ſometimes entirely removes it. This remedy when continued for a ſufficient length of time, ſeems to abate flatulence, to obviate ſpaſm, to improve the appetite, and to ſtrengthen the organs of digeſtion. On theſe tonic powers the virtues of alum muſt chiefly depend; though they may in part ariſe from its obtunding the morbid ſenſibility of the inteſtines, by an immediate action on their nerves.

To

To theſe it is applied more quickly, forcibly, and through a larger extent than moſt other aſtringents, from its ready ſolubility, great ſtypticity, and unchangeable nature. But without diſcuſſing the mode of its operation, I ſhall briefly relate the two following hiſtories, ſelected from ſeveral others, of its ſalutary effects.

CASE I.

January 28th, 1772. Mr. G. aged thirty, a temperate and active man, had been ſubject more than twelve months, to a violent pain in the right *hypogaſtrium,* which often recurred periodically and continued two or three days, leaving a yellowneſs of the countenance, and great ſoreneſs of the *abdomen*. His belly was moderately ſoluble, and his pulſe regular in the ſhort intervals of his fits. For as he lived at a diſtance from Mancheſter, I had no opportunity of ſeeing him in the paroxyſms of his diſorder. The diagnoſtics of this caſe were obſcure, but from a ſuſpicion that his pain might be in the courſe of the ureter, I directed the following medicines.

R. *Pulv. uvæ urſæ ℥j. Aluminis uſti ʒſs. M. f. Pulvis in doſes 24 æquales dividendus; quarum capiat unam ter die, ex unciis tribus decocti ſequentis.*

R. *Rad. petroſelini. paſſular. ſolis. exacinat. aa ℥j. Semin. & ſummit. dauci ſylv. herb. parietar. aa ʒſs. aq. fontanæ ℔iij. coque ad ℔ij. colaturæ & adde ſp. nitri dulcis ʒj. aq. junip. com. ℥iij. M.*

These remedies were continued three weeks, and during the uſe of them the patient ſuffered no return of his diſorder. The medicines proved diuretic, but he diſcharged no gravel, nor did his urine at this time aſſume any remarkable appearance.

Mr.

Mr. G. now conſidered himſelf as cured, and therefore neglected the repetition of his powders. In leſs than a month his cholic recurred with great violence; and, April 27th, 1772, he again applied to me for advice. I preſcribed fifteen grains of burnt alum, and the ſame quantity of ſugar, to be taken twice every day, in any agreeable vehicle, during the ſpace of ſeven or eight weeks. And by ſteadily perſevering in this courſe, he has remained ſix months entirely free from his diſorder.

CASE II.

September 21ſt, 1772. E. P. a houſe-painter, aged 28, had complained ſeveral days of a violent pain in the region of the navel, attended with a ſlight nauſea, and frequent cramps in the extremities. Sixteen hours before I ſaw him he had taken two doſes of caſtor oil, which had yet procured no ſtool, nor afforded any relief. He was now afflicted, during the ſhort remiſſions of his cholic, with very ſevere pains in his arms and ſhoulders. His countenance was yellow; his pulſe beat about ſeventy five ſtrokes in a minute; and his feet were cold. I directed him to go into the warm bath in the evening; and to take the following bolus every ſixth hour.

℞, *Spermatis ceti. aluminis rup. aa* ℈*j. ſyr. ſimplicis q. s. M. f. bolus.*

The pain was much abated by the uſe of this medicine, before he tried the warm bath.

April 27th. He had taken ſeven doſes of alum, and was entirely free from pain; but remained extremely coſtive. The bolus was therefore omitted; and a ſolution of the cathartic ſalt in barley-water was ordered to be given at proper inter-

intervals, till ſeveral ſtools were procured. The ſucceeding day he continued eaſy, but to prevent a relapſe, I preſcribed a ſcruple of alum mixed with an equal quantity of ſugar, to be ſwallowed twice every day, during the following week or fortnight. The patient ſoon recovered his health and ſtrength, and I have reaſon to believe has remained ever ſince free from his diſorder.

CASES

IN WHICH THE

WARM BATH

WAS

SUCCESSFULLY EMPLOYED.

THE uſe of WARM BATHING is of great antiquity. Hippocrates recommends it in the ſtrongeſt terms. *Calidum, ſeu Therma cutim emollit, attenuat, dolores tollit, rigores, convulſiones, nervorum diſtenſiones mitigat, capitis gravitatem ſolvit.* (*a*) Ariſtotle, Pliny, Galen, and Celſus,

(*a*) Hippoc. Aph. 22. Sect. 5.

Celſus, have given their teſtimony in its favour. The Romans derived this practice from the Greeks, and regarded it both as an efficacious remedy, and as one of the higheſt enjoyments of luxury. But under the reign of Auguſtus Cæſar, who was cured of a lingering and dangerous malady, by the uſe of cold bathing, the warm bath fell, for a ſhort time, into diſrepute. This appears from Horace:

Sane Myrteta relinqui
Dictaque ceſſantem nervis elidere morbum
Sulfura contemni; vicus gemit; invidus ægris
Qui caput & ſtomachum ſupponere fontibus audent,
Cluſinis, Gabioſque petunt, & frigida rura.

Hor. Ep. xv.

VAPOUR bathing, as I am well informed, is a univerſal practice amongſt the native Indians of North America. When afflicted with the rheumatiſm, a diſeaſe to which, from their climate, mode of life, and rigid fibres, they are peculiarly incident,

dent, they ſhut themſelves in a cloſe place, and pouring water upon a large ſtone, heated to a ſufficient degree, they expoſe themſelves for a conſiderable time to the ſteams which ariſe from it. Covered with a profuſe ſweat, they then plunge into the cold bath; and afterwards receive the hot vapours as before, repeating for the moſt part twice or thrice theſe ſevere operations. A ſimilar practice prevails in Ruſſia and Siberia; and every perſon in thoſe countries, from the ſovereign, to the meaneſt peaſant, uſes twice in a day ſuch artificial hot baths. The Abbe Chappe d'Auteroche, who travelled into Siberia in the year 1761, by order of the King of France, informs us that the heat of theſe baths is raiſed to 148, and occaſionally even to 168 degrees of Farenheit's thermometer. In this intenſe heat the Ruſſians ſometimes remain two hours, pouring hot water frequently over their bodies; and then ruſh into the open air, diſſolved in ſweat, to roll themſelves in the

the ſnow, during the moſt piercing froſt, when the thermometer ſtands ten degrees below o. Many chronic diſeaſes are cured by this method of bathing; and the rheumatiſm is ſaid to be almoſt unknown in Ruſſia.

Prosper Alpinus relates that warm baths are uſed by the Egyptians, in all fevers except thoſe of the peſtilential kind; and in a variety of other diſorders. They are employed alſo by the females of that country, eſpecially by the Hebrew women, to render them more corpulent. "*Quod ut obtineant, multis diebus, dulcibus tepidis Balneis indulgent, in ijſque diu morantes, comedunt, potant, clyſteribuſque ibi ex variis pinguedinibus, ac adipibus paratis utuntur, multaque etiam medicamenta per os aſſumunt.*

In England warm bathing is rarely employed in private practice, notwithſtanding ſeveral modern writers of reputation

tation have ſtrongly recommended it; and the experience of ages hath evinced its utility. To excite more attention to a remedy, which though well known is too much neglected, I ſhall briefly relate a few caſes in which it proved eminently ſucceſsful.

CASE I.

January 14th, 1770. A young gentleman, of an irritable habit, after drinking freely and ſwallowing a large quantity of Cayenne pepper, was ſeized with an inflammatory *angina*. The fever, ſwelling of the *fauces*, laborious reſpiration, difficult deglution, and violent pain in the head, were ſucceeded by a delirium; and although theſe ſymptoms were in ſome degree mitigated by venæſection, cathartics, bliſters, leeches applied to the throat, *pediluvia*, and by nitrous and antimonial medicines, yet they continued with great ſeverity,

ſeverity, and the patient paſſed ſix days and nights without enjoying the leaſt ſlumber. Under theſe circumſtances (January 20th) the warm bath was preſcribed, and the young gentleman directed to ſit in it half an hour. The delirium ſoon abated; he fell into a profound and refreſhing ſleep, in which he continued thirteen hours; and then awoke entirely free from fever or delirium. And in a ſhort time he recovered his uſual health and ſtrength.

CASE II.

MASTER S. P. aged two years, healthy but of a delicate make, and with a head larger than is natural, was ſeized Auguſt 13th, 1771, at one o'clock in the morning, with ſevere convulſions. He had been ſlightly indiſpoſed a day or two before, and the preceding evening a few eruptions were obſerved on his face and neck.

neck. His ſiſter was juſt recovered from the ſmall pox, and he had not been ſeparated from her during her illneſs, ſo that there remained no doubt concerning the cauſe of theſe ſymptoms. An emetic was adminiſtered, and a laxative clyſter afterwards injected. But the fits continued with great violence, recurring at ſhorter and ſhorter intervals, notwithſtanding the application of a bliſter to the back, an antiſpaſmodic liniment to the ſpine, and the aſſiduous uſe of paregoric elixir, fœtid *ſal volatile*, muſk, camphor, the *pediluvium*, &c. The child's ſtrength was now almoſt exhauſted, his reſpiration became laborious, his extremities cold, his pulſe trembling, quick and languid, and his face was alternately fluſhed, and of a cadaverous paleneſs. The variolous eruption neither increaſed nor receded.

Such was the ſituation of my little patient at eleven o'clock at night, when I directed him to be immerſed, as high

as

as the chin, in warm water. The relief this afforded was almoſt inſtantaneous. Every convulſive motion ceaſed, his breathing became free and regular, he took notice of thoſe around him, and ſeemed ſenſible of the preſent eaſe he enjoyed. He remained in the bath about ten minutes, and was much refreſhed by it, but had a fit not long afterwards: This however was very ſlight, and yielded immediately to a clyſter prepared of a ſtrong infuſion of Valerian root and aſſafætida, with a few drops of tinct. Thebaica which was in readineſs, and ſhould have been injected on his coming out of the water. He retained the clyſter only a few minutes, but paſſed the reſt of the night in a compoſed and comfortable ſleep, and the next morning the eruption was univerſal. The puſtules were diſtinct, but ſo ſlow in ſuppurating, that they died away without coming to any degree of maturity, although a cordial diet was enjoined, the bark preſcribed, and ſmall doſes of ſulphur, mixed with ſyrup of poppies, were frequently adminiſtered.

CASE III.

Mrs. H. aged thirty-five, a lady of a tender conſtitution, ſubject to ſcorbutic eruptions, and enfeebled by frequent child bearing, received in the beginning of January 1770, a ſevere ſhock by the untimely death of an infant at the breaſt, which occaſioned a miſcarriage and profuſe uterine hæmorrhage. A variety of hyſterical ſymptoms ſucceeded, and gradually increaſed. February 18th, my aſſiſtance was deſired. She was then afflicted with great languor of body, and dejection of mind, with flatulence, want of appetite, and a violent ſenſe of ſuffocation in her throat. Every morning a *delirium* came on, attended with ſevere convulſions. Her pulſe was quick, fluttering, and irregular; her ſkin was dry,

and

and ſince her miſcarriage free from any eruption; and ſhe complained of an oppreſſion about the *præcordia*. A bliſter, to the head was directed; a cordial and nouriſhing diet recommended; and the frequent uſe of the *pediluvium* enjoined. The following medicines were alſo preſcribed.

℞. *Aſſafœtidæ electæ gr. xv. Pulv. Ipecac. extract. Thebaic. aa gr. j. Ol. Menthæ gutt. ij. ſyr. ſimp. q. s. M. f. Pilulæ mediocres omni nocte hora ſomni ſumendæ.*

℞. *Pulv. Cort. Peruvian. ʒj. Raſur. Ligni Guaiac. Saſafras, Cort. Winteran. Rad. Glycyrrhiz. aa ʒij. Aq. Font. bullient. ℔j. Infunde, vaſe clauſo per ſex horas, deinde cola.*

℞. *Colaturæ præſcriptæ ℥iſs. Tinct Valerian. vol. Tinct. Caſtor. aa ʒj. M. f. Hauſtus ter die ſumendus.*

 BY

By theſe remedies ſhe was much relieved, and continued better till the 12th of March; when ſhe relapſed into all her former complaints, which recurred with an increaſed degree of dejection and anxiety of mind. Without my knowledge ſhe had tried the cold bath, and had been ſenſibly injured by it. No eruption yet appeared on her ſkin; and the delirium, which was more violent than before, now invaded her always in the evening. Troches of ſulphur and the compound lime water, with the pills mentioned above were at this time preſcribed; and the patient was directed to uſe the warm bath every night, previous to the aceeſſion of the delirium.

March 13th. The delirium recurred with much leſs violence, and was of ſhorter continuance; and after bathing the patient fell into a ſound and compoſed ſleep.

March 16th. The warm bath was omitted, and the delirium was much more violent,

violent, and lafted longer. The following draught was directed to be taken an hour before its acceffion, the fucceeding evening, and the ufe of the bath to be repeated.

R. *Sagapeni, Mofch. aa gr. x. Camphoræ gr. ij. Mucilag. Gum. Arab. q. s. fimul tritis gradatim adde Aquæ Menth. vulg. fimp.* ℥ *ifs. Tinct. Valer. fimp.* ʒ *ij. Syr. è Cort. Aurant.* ʒ *j. M. f. Hauftus.*

By thefe means, affiduoufly purfued, the patient recovered her health before the end of March. Whenever the warm bath was omitted, which happened twice or thrice, fhe fuffered fenfibly by the neglect. Her delirium was more fevere, and of longer duration, her fleep was fhorter and lefs refrefhing, and the fucceeding day fhe was more troubled with anxiety of mind, oppreffion about the *præcordia*, and other nervous fymptoms.

CASE IV.

A LEARNED and very benevolent clergyman, who resides about forty miles from Manchester, consulted me by letter in the beginning of March, 1769. He had been several years afflicted with a variety of hypochondriacal complaints, which had succeeded the sudden repulsion of an eruption on his foot, by means of an astringent bath; and he was then under a continual anxiety and distraction of mind. He had one prevailing idea constantly in his head, and one distressing image before his eyes. These symptoms of his disorder he ascribed to a violent commotion of mind, at a time when he was under great depression of spirits, and which occasioned a sudden start, or convulsive motion, in one part of his head. In this part he felt a constant and forcible spasm, which he supposed extended itself

to

to his breaſt and bowels, as he generally perceived a ſenſe of contraction in thoſe parts, attended with an inward heat. His eyes were particularly affected, being drawn as it were out of their ſockets, and endued with an unnatural ſenſibility. In a ſecond letter dated March 11th, he informed me that he perceived every night, when he lay in bed, a continual motion from his forehead upwards, and about his temples, like the undulation of waves. The uneaſineſs and pain in his head was ſo extreme, that he could not bear even the preſſure of his hat. But all this bodily pain was trifling in degree when compared to the diſtreſs of his mind, ariſing from the irreſiſtible force with which external objects diſtracted his eyes and imagination.

UNDER theſe unhappy circumſtances he had conſulted ſeveral Phyſicians of great eminence, and had tried a variety of medicines, the detail of which, as well as of thoſe which I preſcribed to him, would be equally tedious and unneceſſary. Nothing had afforded him ſo much relief as the warm *pediluvium*, and the extract of opium, of which he had habituated himſelf to take ten or twelve grains every day. Medicine proving ſo ineffectual, I adviſed the gradual diſcontinuance of his opiates; recommended the frequent uſe of the warm bath; and directed hot water to be poured in a ſtream, upon the part of his head which was moſt affected. The following paſſages extracted from his letters, ſhew the beneficial conſequences of this courſe. "My days begin to be eaſier, and I have not had ſuch bad nights ſince I went into the warm bath, which is near two months ago. It has wonderfully ſoftened and compoſed my head, and enabled me to ſleep ſooner and ſounder than I uſed to do. I have made ſeveral attempts to uſe the cold bath along with it, but I am always obliged to deſiſt, as

it

it immediately alters me for the worſe, greatly increaſes the diſtreſs in my head, and renders my ſleep more diſturbed. I am however attempting it again; and I hope with a better proſpect of ſucceſs. I ſhould be much encouraged by finding myſelf able to bear it; as I am perſuaded it would have a happy effect in ſtrengthening and reſtoring me."—" I find myſelf daily advancing towards a more perfect ſtate of health. I have brought myſelf at length to bear the cold bath very well. I uſe it every other day, and find a very happy effect from it, in reſtoring my ſpirits and ſtrengthening my whole frame. But it would not do without the aſſiſtance of the warm bath, which is my conſtant antidote againſt any diſagreeable effects from the other, and gives me never failing relief and reſt at night. The pouring warm water, in a conſtant ſtream, upon that part of my head, where my complaint lies, has I apprehend, been of ſingular ſervice in ſoftening and opening it, and

and contributed greatly to that happy change which I find in myſelf. I have been gradually weaning myſelf from opium; and have reduced the doſe from three pills to one."

This gentleman ſoon recovered his health, and has been ever ſince free from any returns of his diſorder.

I have recommended warm bathing in a variety of other complaints, and for the moſt part with the happieſt ſucceſs. Like other remedies, however, it has ſometimes diſappointed my expectations; and in two inſtances its operation proved in ſome degree unfavourable. The one caſe was a violent pain reſembling the ſciatica, but which I believe proceeded from an affection of the kidney. The other was a moſt troubleſome ſenſe of motion in the *uterus* from one ſide of the pelvis to the other, which occurred at the end of of every fortnight, in the intervals between the *catamenia*, and lasted generally three or four days. The patient was free from this complaint when in a sitting posture; and it was most uneasy to her when she was walking. The warm bath aggravated the pain in the former instance; and seemed to protract the disorder a day or two in the latter.

MIS-

MISCELLANEOUS

C A S E S

A N D

O B S E R V A T I O N S.

1. IT is highly probable that Palsies frequently arise from diseases of the *viscera*, without any previous fault in the brain or spinal marrow. And considerable errors may be committed in practice, by a want of precision in distinguishing the

the causes from which they proceed. Large evacuations are often indiscriminately directed in these disorders, from a supposition that they arise from plenitude; and thus irreparable mischief is done in those cases of weakness or irritability, which are now most numerous.

I HAVE seen several *hemiplegias* which derived their origin from affections of the liver; others from an *atonia* of the stomach and bowels; and three instances have occurred to me of Palsies from pregnancy. The following history is of this kind.

MRS. D. of Rochdale, aged 21, whose *menses* had always recurred with regularity, but attended with great pain and general disorder, in the spring of 1771 had a miscarriage. The following August the *catamenia* did not appear at the usual period. She had a violent pain in the loins and about the *os sacrum*, which continued

tinued ſeveral hours, and was then ſucceeded by a pain equally acute in her head. Soon afterwards ſhe loſt all power of ſpeech, and the uſe of her right ſide. Her habit was not plethoric, but an experienced and ſenſible Apothecary, before my arrival, had taken from her arm half a pound of blood, had applied a bliſter to her back, and a volatile liniment to the ſide affected. By theſe means ſhe recovered in about ſixteen hours the uſe of her ſide, but ſtill complained of a *torpor* in it, and of a dull pain and confuſion in her head. Her pulſe was ſoft and natural, and her blood of a proper texture. I conſidered the palſy as ariſing from an uterine affection; and directed a gentle purgative of rhubarb and magneſia every other night, and an infuſion of Peruvian bark and Valerian, to ſtrengthen the habit of the patient, and to abate irritability. Venæſection was alſo recommended a few days before the next period of the *catamenia*. At the return of this

this period ſhe had a ſecond paralytic ſtroke, of the ſame kind as before, and preceded by the like ſymptoms. Venæſection had been omitted, and ſhe had neglected her medicines. She was now evidently in a ſtate of pregnancy. I adviſed a repetition of the remedies before preſcribed; and recommended the uſe of a temperately cold bath. She cemplied with theſe injunctions, and had no return of her diſorder.

2. FULLER, in his *Medicina Gymnaſtica*, ſtrongly recommends COLTSFOOT in conſumptive diſorders. It appears to be anodyne and a corrector of acrimony; but only exerts theſe powers when taken in a large quantity. I gave a ſtrong infuſion of it to a young woman, who had various running ſores, hectic heats, a colliquative *diarrhœa*, and wandering pains all over her body. It produced a better digeſtion in the ulcers, alleviated her pains, and abated the violence of the *diarrhœa*.

diarrhœa. Cicuta, and Peruvian bark were before adminiſtered with good effect, but had been for ſome time diſcontinued, on account of their expenſiveneſs. I thought the *tupilago* afforded more relief to the patient than either of them.

3. LARGE doſes of opium have been frequently adminiſtered in painful and ſpaſmodic diſeaſes, not only with ſafety, but with the happieſt ſucceſs. A very learned and ingenious practitioner informs me that he lately gave to a lady in the fifth month of her pregnancy, who had an acute pain in her bowels, which threatened an abortion, twenty-two grains of the extract of opium, and three hundred drops of laudanum, in the ſpace of thirty-ſix hours. And by theſe means, and theſe alone, ſhe perfectly recovered. But the nervous ſyſtem, eſpecially in ſpaſmodic diſorders, is ſubject to great and ſudden changes, which muſt ſometimes render the doſes of medicines, powerful in their

their operation, uncertain and liable to produce the moſt dangerous effects. The following caſe, communicated to me by a young phyſician, who is likely to be an ornament to his profeſſion, affords a ſtriking confirmation of the truth of this obſervation.

A YOUTH, who was admitted into the hoſpital at —— on account of a violent ſpaſmodic diſeaſe, which recurred periodically in the evening, after trying a variety of remedies, was directed to take the *extractum Thebaicum* in ſuch a quantity as might prove ſufficient to mitigate the violence of the paroxyſms. The doſe amounted to twenty-two grains, and was repeated every night, during the ſpace of a week, without producing any ſoporific effects. On the eighth night it was obſerved that he had no return of the ſpaſm; and in the morning he was found dead. It is probable that a ſudden alteration had taken place in the nervous ſyſtem of this

 patient,

patient, and that the opium, in conſequence of it, exerted with full force its uſual powers on the body.

4. I HAVE lately received from a clergyman of great learning and humanity, a ſmall quantity of ſeed, which is brought from the coaſt of Malabar, and is celebrated in the Eaſt Indies as a powerful remedy for the cholic. It is called by the Portugueſe AJAVA. " Captain B. formerly commander of the Prince Henry Indiaman, procured ſome of it from the Jeſuit's College at Goa, brought it over with him to England, and diſtributed it amongſt ſuch of his neighbours and acquaintance as were troubled with the cholic, who found great benefit from the uſe of it. Being himſelf exceedingly afflicted at times with the windy gout, and having in one of his fits applied ſeveral things in vain, he made trial of the *ajava ſeed*, and found it ſo very efficacious in expelling the wind, and removing the gout

gout from the ſtomach and head, that he has ever ſince taken it on the like occaſions. The moſt uſual effect of it is to procure a plentiful diſcharge of wind, and ſometimes it relieves the diſorder by a ſtool or two." From the ſenſible qualities of this ſeed, I ſhould judge it to be an active remedy: But I have yet had no experience of its efficacy, and I mention it only to promote an enquiry into its medicinal virtues.

5. A LADY, aged 40, was ſubject ſeveral years to an exceſſive degree of acidity in her ſtomach and bowels, which medicines ſometimes palliated, but never cured. By degrees the acidity abated, and at length entirely ceaſed; but ſhe became ſubject to frequent diarrhœas, to a *profluvium menſium*, and to copious and ſudden diſcharges of urine. She complained of great feebleneſs, of wearineſs in her legs, and of a conſtant pain in her loins. Her pulſe was languid and ſlow,

her ſkin cold, of a dark hue, and covered with freckles. She had often a putrid taſte in her mouth, at which time the ſaliva was tinged with blood; and in the intervals of her *menſes* ſhe had a continual diſcharge of brown, fœtid water from the *uterus*.

THESE ſymptoms are characteriſtics of a true ſcurvy or diſſolution of the blood; which in this inſtance ſeems to have been produced by the long continuance of an acid acrimony in the firſt paſſages. Dr. Gaubius has well deſcribed the effects of ſuch an acrimony. *Acor primis maxime viis infeſtus, tempore & ſanguinem humoreſque inde deductos ſubiens, naſcitur ex uſu diuturno acidorum aut aceſcentium, quæ viribus corporis non ſubiguntur; aut quia ex ſe indomabilia ſunt naturæ humanæ, aut ob virtutis coctricis impotentiam. Debilitas igitur ſolidorum univerſalis, aut privata viſcerum primæ digeſtionis; irritabilitas regulares horum motus turbans; inertia defectuſve ſuccorum præ-*

præparantium; circulationis & caloris naturalis languor; neglectus motus animalis, eo disponunt, ut pateat, cui maxime ætati, sexui, vitæ generi, hoc acre frequentius eveniat. (*a*)

To determine the comparative nutritive powers of different foods, a few years ago a Physician, of distinguished abilities, made a variety of experiments, to which he at length fell an unfortunate sacrifice. I have been well informed that he lived a month upon bread and water only, by which he daily diminished in his weight. At the end of that time, he added sugar to his bread and water, and confined himself a fortnight longer to this diet. His breath then became offensive, his gums bled, putrid sloughs appeared in his mouth, and *vibices* spread themselves over different parts of his body. These symptoms were removed by a return to animal diet, and by the use of the bark.

(*a*) Gaubij Pathologia, Sect. 307.

It is contrary to the prevailing THEORY, that vegetable food ſhould give riſe to putrefaction in the animal ſyſtem; but there are many proofs of the truth of it. Doctor Biſſet relates ſeveral caſes of highly putrid fevers, quick in their progreſs and fatal in their termination, wherein the ſeptic ferment evidently began in the *primæ viæ* after eating heartily of aceſcent food. Calves alſo put to graze in a rich paſture, towards the cloſe of autumn, are ſometimes affected with a putrid diſeaſe, which deſtroys them in thirty hours. The farmers call it the *quarter felon*, becauſe one hind quarter becomes putrid and emphyſematous; and as ſoon as the *emphyſema* extends to the ſpine, the animal expires: It is moſt incident to calves that are healthy. Juices, which are perfectly animalized or aſſimilated, are leſs prone to putrefy than ſuch as are crude, or blended with a great proportion of aceſcent chyle. The meat of bullocks and of ſheep which have been kept faſting a ſufficient

ſufficient length of time before they are killed, that is till the recent chyle be completely aſſimilated, is firmer and continues ſweet much longer, than the fleſh of ſuch as are ſlaughtered ſoon after taking them from their paſtures. *(b)*

THE learned writer whom I have quoted above obſerves. *Dulciaria, ſaccharata, mellita, hiſque ſimilia, uſu immodico, per occultam acrimoniam dentibus inimica ſunt; pro vi ſua fermentante, acidum ingenerant, et quæ ex hoc profluunt mala; præterea ſolvunt tenuantque humores; horum minuta denſitate et firmas partes relaxant; non uno hinc nomine generi nervoſo infeſta, infantibus, ſexui ſequiori, debilibus, hyſtericis, hypochondriacis, obſunt.* *(c)*

FROM the uſeful and accurate experiments of Sir John Pringle it appears that

 bread,

(b) Vid. Biſſet's Medical Obſervations, p. 85.

(c) Gaubij Pathologia, Sect. 470.

bread, water, and fresh gall, when fermented together, first turned sour, then putrid. And Doctor Bryan Robinson found that perspiration is diminished by fruit, and garden vegetables. Perhaps these facts may reflect some light on the preceding observations.

6. Mr. William White of York, the ingenious author of an Essay on the Diseases of the Bile, has lately communicated to me some curious experiments on the solution of those calculous concretions, which are called gall stones. He has discovered that *alcohol* saturated with *oleum terebinthinæ æthereum*, quickly and totally dissolves them. And induced by the powerful action of this *menstruum* out of the body, he has administered it internally with some degree of success; and is desirous of recommending it to the trial of others. Such a remedy, if it prove effectual, must be regarded as a valuable addition to the *materia medica*. But if we consider

consider the peculiar œconomy observed by nature in the circulation of the blood through the liver; the long stagnation of the bile in the gall bladder; and the quickness with which *alcohol* and oil of turpentine pass off by urine and perspiration, it is to be feared that such a *menstruum*, powerful as it may be, will scarcely reach the solvend. To this objection also we may add, that the diagnostics of the disease are often obscure and uncertain. The same gentleman informs me, that he was not long since present at the dissection of a woman, who had laboured several months under an obstinate jaundice, attended with violent and periodical pains in the region of the liver, with costiveness, white stools, and other symptoms of biliary concretions. No such cause however was found; but a large schirrus, extended itself from the *pylorus* along the *duodenum*, so as to close the orifice of the *ductus communis*, and thus prevent the passage of the bile into the intestines. But

I mean

I mean not to diſcourage, and wiſh rather to promote the trial of a medicine, which is active in its properties, and yet unlikely to prove injurious in its operation. Such experiments are juſtified by a maxim well known, and of undoubted authority in phyſic.

7. I COMMUNICATED ſome time ago to Doctor Prieſtley, the hiſtory of a putrid fever, in which the injection of mephitic air into the inteſtines, was attended with very beneficial effects. The Doctor has annexed it to his papers on factitious air, which will probably be publiſhed in the next volume of the Philoſophical Tranſactions. A caſe, of the ſame kind, has very lately occurred to me; and I ſhall here briefly relate the moſt important particulars of it.

ELIZABETH GRUNDY, aged ſeventeen, was attacked on the 16th of December, 1772, with the uſual ſymptoms of a continued

tinued fever: The common method of cure was purſued; but the diſeaſe increaſed, and ſoon aſſumed a putrid type. On the 23d, I found her labouring under a conſtant *delirium*, with a *ſubſultus tendinum*: Her ſkin was hot and dry, her tongue black, her thirſt immoderate, and her ſtools were frequent, extremely offenſive, and for the moſt part involuntary. Her pulſe beat about 130 ſtrokes in a minute; ſhe doſed much; and was very deaf. I directed wine to be adminiſtered freely; a bliſter to be applied to her back; the *pediluvium* to be uſed ſeveral times in the day; and mephitic air to be injected, under the form of a clyſter, every two hours. The next day her ſtools were leſs frequent, had loſt their fœtor, and were no longer diſcharged involuntarily; her pulſe was reduced to 110 ſtrokes in a minute; and her *delirium* was much abated. Directions were given to repeat the clyſters, and to ſupply the patient liberally with wine. Theſe means were aſſiduouſly

ously purſued ſeveral days; and the young woman was ſo much recruited by the 28th, that the injection was diſcontinued. She was now quite rational, and not averſe to medicine: A decoction of the Peruvian bark was therefore preſcribed; by the uſe of which ſhe ſpeedily recovered her health.

PRO-

PROPOSALS

FOR ESTABLISHING MORE

ACCURATE AND COMPREHENSIVE

BILLS

OF

MORTALITY.

Fluminis ritu feruntur.

Hor.

Fas eſt et ab hoſte doceri.

Ovid. Metam.

PROPOSALS FOR ESTABLISHING MORE ACCURATE AND COMPREHENSIVE BILLS OF MORTALITY IN MANCHESTER.

THE eſtabliſhment of a judicious and accurate regiſter of the births and burials, in every town and pariſh, would be attended with the moſt important advantages, medical, political, and moral. By ſuch an inſtitution, the increaſe or decreaſe of certain diſeaſes; the comparative healthineſs of different ſituations, climates, and ſeaſons; the influence of particular trades and manufactures on longevity; with many other curious circumſtances, not more intereſting to Phyſicians.

ſicians, than beneficial to mankind, would be aſcertained with tolerable preciſion. In a political view, exact regiſters of human mortality are of ſtill greater conſequence, as the number of people and the progreſs of population in the kingdom, may in the moſt eaſy and unexceptionable manner, be deduced from them. They are the foundation likewiſe of all calculations concerning the values of aſſurances on lives, reverſionary payments, and of every ſcheme for providing annuities for widows, and perſons in old age. In a moral light alſo ſuch *tables* are of evident utility, as the increaſe of vice or virtue may be determined, by obſerving the proportion which the diſeaſes ariſing from luxury, intemperance, and other ſimilar cauſes bear to the reſt; and in what particular places diſtempers of this claſs are found to be moſt fatal.

A FEW examples may perhaps confirm and illuſtrate theſe obſervations. In the Pais

Pais de Vaud, a diſtrict of the province of Bern in Switzerland, and in a country pariſh in Brandenburgh, 1 in 45 of the inhabitants die annually;. and at Stoke Damarell in Devonſhire, 1 in 54; whereas in Vienna, and Edinburgh, the yearly mortality appears to be 1 in 20; in London 1 in 21; in Amſterdam and Rome 1 in 22; in Northampton 1 in 26; and in the pariſh of Holy Croſs, near Shrewſbury, 1 in 33. In the Pais de Vaud, the proportion of inhabitants who attain the age of eighty, is 1 in 21½; in Brandenburgh 1 in 22½; in Norwich 1 in 27; in Mancheſter 1 in 30; in London 1 in 40; and in Edinburgh 1 in 42. Theſe facts afford a ſtriking but melancholy proof, of the unfavourable influence of large towns on the duration of life.—From the moſt accurate computation, London is found to contain 601750 inhabitants; and from 1759 to 1768, the burials have exceeded the chriſtenings every year upwards of 7000; which is the recruit the metropolis requires annually from the country, to ſupport the preſent number of its people. In 1757, a ſurvey was made of Mancheſter and Salford. The number of inhabitants then amounted to 19839; and the burials, excluſive of thoſe amongſt Diſſenters, were 778. But ſince that time the populouſneſs of Mancheſter has conſiderably increaſed. Half of all that are born in this town die under five years old. The iſland of Madeira is ſo remarkably healthy, that two thirds of all who are born in it live to be married. Autumn is the moſt healthy, and ſummer the moſt ſickly ſeaſon there. The mortality of ſpring and ſummer, is to that of autumn and winter, as 115 to 100. In Mancheſter, diſeaſes are moſt frequent and fatal in the months of January, February, and March; and leaſt ſo in July, Auguſt, and September. The mortality of theſe two ſeaſons is as 11 to 8; and of the

the firſt ſix months of the year, compared with the laſt ſix months, as 7 to 6. M. Muret, Secretary to the Oeconomical Society at Bern, informs us, that he had the curioſity to examine the regiſter of mortality in one town, and to mark thoſe whoſe deaths might be imputed to intemperance. And he found the number ſo great, as to incline him to believe that drunkenneſs is more deſtructive to mankind than pleuriſies, fevers, or the moſt malignant diſtempers. *(a)* Such are the important uſes, to which Tables of Human Mortality have been applied.

THE following plan of a more exact and comprehenſive regiſter, than has hitherto been kept, is ſubmitted to the conſideration and correction of thoſe who

(a) Vid. a very valuable Treatiſe on Reverſionary Payments, by the Rev. Dr. Price; the Bern Obſervations for the year 1766; Philoſophical Tranſactions, vol. 57 and 59; and Dr. Short's new Obſervations.

undertake the charge of the BILLS of MORTALITY in *Manchefter*.

1. LET a table of *chriftenings*, *marriages*, and *burials* be kept in every church, chapel, and place of religious worfhip in the town, and delivered at certain ftated times, to the clerk of the parifh church, to be formed into one general BILL, and quarterly or annually publifhed. It is of importance that the *ftill born* children, and thofe who die before *baptifm*, fhould alfo be regiftered; and the midwives fhould be defired to deliver an account of them. Perhaps the fextons may affift in afcertaining their number, as they are ufually interred in church yards, or other public burial grounds.

2. LET the table of *chriftenings* fpecify the *males* and *females* who are baptized; and the table of *deaths* exprefs the *males* who die, under the feveral denominations of

of children, batchelors, married men, and widowers; the *females* who die under the correſponding denominations of children, maidens, married women, and widows. An obſervance of theſe diſtinctions will determine the comparative number of *males* and *females* who are born; the difference between the ſexes in the expectation of life; and the proportion which the annual births, deaths, and marriages bear to each other. Thus by the BILLS of MORTALITY which have been kept at Vienna, Breſlaw, Dreſden, Leipſic, Ratiſbon, and other towns in Germany, it appears that the proportion of *males* to the *females* who are born is as 19 to 18: But the proportion of *boys* to *girls* who die under ten years of age, is as 7 to 6; and of *married men* to *married women* in Breſlaw as 5 to 3; in Dreſden as 4 to 1. At Vevey, in Switzerland, for 20 years, ending in 1764, there died in the firſt month 135, *males* to 89 *females*; and in the first year 225, to 162. The same accounts shew likewise that both at Vevey and Berlin, the *still-born males* are to the *still-born females* as 30 to 21. In the parish of Holy Cross, Salop, an account was taken by the Vicar, A. D. 1760, of the number of *males* and *females* of the age of seventy and upwards: The latter amounted to *thirty-five*, the former only to *eight*. At Paris, and in Sweden, it has been observed, that *women* not only live longer than *men*, but that *married women* live longer than *single women*. And in Switzerland it appears particularly, from the calculations of M. Muret, that of equal numbers of *single* and *married* women, between the age of 15 and 25, more of the former died than of the latter, in the proportion of 2 to 1. *(b)*

3. Let the ages of the dead under *five*,

(b) Vid. Dr. Price's Observations on Reversionary Payments.

five, be ſpecified by ſingle years; and afterwards, by periods of five or ten years.

4. LET the BILLS of MORTALITY contain not only a liſt of the diſeaſes of which all die, but alſo expreſs particularly, the number dying of each diſeaſe, in the ſeveral diviſions of life and different ſeaſons of the year. To accompliſh this it will be neceſſary for the Phyſicians of the town, to conſider the preſent liſt of diſtempers; to reject all ſynonymous and obſolete terms; and to give a ſhort and eaſy explanation of thoſe which are retained. And whenever a perſon dies, who has been attended by any of the faculty, the Phyſician, Surgeon, or Apothecary, ſhould be deſired to certify in writing the age, and diſtemper of the deceaſed.

THE following TABLES are conſtructed upon this PLAN; and if the ſcale be

 enlarged,

enlarged, will ſerve for the *Church Regiſter*, as well as for quarterly or annual publication. It appears to be unneceſſary, and in many inſtances would be exceptionable, to inſert the names of the deceaſed: Their *denomination* and *diſeaſe* therefore, may be expreſſed, in the columns allotted to each, by dots or units, which are to be ſummed up at the end of every three months, and ſet down in figures.

THE LISTS of *Marriages* and *Chriſtenings* may be kept in the common method.

THE additional trouble which this more comprehenſive and accurate REGISTER will occaſion to the Clerks of the ſeveral churches, &c. may be compenſated by diſtributing amongſt them, at the diſcretion of any judicious clergyman, the money which ariſes from the ſale of the quarterly BILLS. If a hundred of theſe

theſe be ſubſcribed for, or ſold at the price of one ſhilling each, the ſum of twenty pounds per annum will thus be raiſed, without impoſing any new burthens on the town. Every ſecond, third, fourth, or fifth year the bills may be collected into a volume, and publiſhed, under the direction of two or more Phyſicians, with obſervations on the ſtate of the weather, the prevalence of epidemic diſeaſes, their ſymptoms and method of cure, and the increaſe or decreaſe of population during that period. Such a work will afford the moſt important inſtruction to the public; and from the profits of it, a fund may be eſtabliſhed for the benefit of the Clerks, and the ſupport of the inſtitution.

N. B. It is obvious that the plan here propoſed is not local, and that it may be executed with equal facility and advantage in every town and pariſh in the

the kingdom.—BILLS of MORTALITY might be rendered more uſeful in a political view, by taking ſometimes the number of houſes and inhabitants, under and above particular ages,. wherever ſuch regiſters are eſtabliſhed.

TABLE

L

TABLE of DEATHS.

January, February, March.

Ages.	Males.	Females.	Ages.	Batchelors.	Married Men.	Widowers.	Maidens.	Married Wo-menl	Widows.
1.			20.						
2.			25.						
3.			30.						
4.			35.						
5.			40.						
10.			45.						
15.			50.						
Total under 15.			60.						
			&c. &c.						

TABLE of DISEASES.

January, February, March.

DISEASES.	1.	2.	3	4.	5.	10.	20.	30.	40.	50.	60.	70.	80.	90.	100.	
Casualties.																
Apoplexy.																
Asthma.																
Cancer.																
Chincough.																
Cholic.																
Consumption.																
Convulsions.																
&c. &c.																

A GENERAL

INDEX.

A.

Buxton

Chamomile

F.

H.

Hiſtory,

Nitrous

N.

O.

P.

Salep

S.

Salt,

Warm

THE END.

E R R A T A.

In various places for *hæmorrhage* read *hæmorrhage*.

Page.	Line.	
13,	3,	for *are* read *is*.
33,	last,	for *indiſpoſed* read *not diſpoſed*.
43,	6,	for *beat up* read *beaten*.
46,	9,	for *draft* read *draff*.
72,	9,	for *thirty* read *twenty*.
105,	2,	for *haſted* read *haſtened*.
116,	12,	for *minute* read *ſmall*.
125,	11,	for *beat* read *beaten*.
185,	9,	for *chorea ſ. vitæ* read *chorea S. V*iii.
224,	9,	for *tupilago* read *tuſſilago*.

Printed in the United States
By Bookmasters